INTERMITTENT

FASTING

SOLUTIONS

FOR

WOMEN OVER 50

TRANSFORM YOUR HEALTH: SHED POUNDS, SLOW AGING, BOOST ENERGY, ENHANCE WELL-BEING, AND SAVOR LIFE

BROOKLYN LUCAS

This book is designed for educational and informational purposes only. The content aims to enhance understanding and appreciation of health-related topics. Any references to specific events, names, or copyrighted materials are included for commentary, criticism, or review.

The author and publisher are not responsible for any negative effects that may arise, directly or indirectly, from the information provided in this book.

TABLE OF CONTENT

INTRODUCTION

As women, our bodies undergo incredible transformations throughout our lives. The transition into our 50s marks another significant phase, one filled with both challenges and opportunities. This book, "Intermittent Fasting Solutions for Women Over 50: Transform Your Health: Shed Pounds, Slow Aging, Boost Energy, Enhance Well-Being, and Savor Life," is dedicated to empowering you to embrace this new chapter with confidence and grace.

The idea of intermittent fasting might seem daunting at first, especially with all the changes that come with age. But intermittent fasting is not just a diet; it's a lifestyle that has the potential to revolutionize your health and well-being. This book is your comprehensive guide to understanding and implementing intermittent fasting in a way that aligns with your unique needs as a woman over 50.

In the pages that follow, you will discover the science behind intermittent fasting, tailored specifically to address the hormonal shifts and metabolic changes that occur as we age. You'll learn practical strategies to start and sustain a fasting routine, along with delicious recipes and meal plans designed to nourish your body and support your fasting journey. We'll also elaborate the importance of exercise, stress management, and emotional well-being, providing you with a holistic approach to health.

Let me share with you the story of Karen, a vibrant 55-year-old woman who transformed her life through intermittent fasting and a holistic approach to health. Karen had always been active, but as she entered her 50s, she began to experience unexplained weight gain, fatigue, and mood swings. She tried various diets and exercise routines, but nothing seemed to work long-term. Feeling frustrated and defeated, Karen stumbled upon the concept of intermittent fasting.

Karen decided to give it a try, starting with a simple 16/8 fasting schedule—fasting for 16 hours and eating within an 8-hour window. She focused on eating nutrient-dense foods and incorporated regular exercise into her routine. But Karen didn't stop there; she also embraced mindfulness practices, meditation, and yoga to manage stress and enhance her emotional well-being.

Within a few weeks, Karen noticed significant changes. She started shedding pounds, her energy levels soared, and her mood stabilized. Her friends and family were amazed at her transformation. Karen felt like she had found a new lease on life. Intermittent fasting, combined with a holistic approach to health, had not only improved her physical health but also her mental and emotional well-being.

Karen's story is just one example of the incredible benefits that intermittent fasting can offer. This book will provide you with all the tools, knowledge, and inspiration you need to embark on your own journey towards better health. Whether you're looking to lose weight, boost your energy, slow down aging, or simply enhance your overall well-being, intermittent fasting can be the key to unlocking your full potential.

As you read through this book, remember that this journey is about more than just fasting; it's about embracing a healthier, more fulfilling life. Together, we will explore the power of intermittent fasting and holistic health, and you'll find that it's never too late to transform your health and savor life to the fullest.

CHAPTER ONE

EMBRACING A NEW JOURNEY

"The only journey is the one within." – Rainer Maria Rilke

As women, we often spend our lives caring for others, nurturing our families, and building our careers. By the time we reach our 50s, we may find that we have put our own needs and health on the back burner. This stage of life, however, offers a unique opportunity for self-care and transformation. The body's needs change as we age, and what worked in our 20s or 30s might no longer be effective. Intermittent fasting, an age-old practice that has gained renewed attention in recent years, can be a powerful tool for women over 50 to embrace a new journey toward optimal health.

Intermittent fasting is not just another diet trend; it's a lifestyle change that can lead to significant health benefits. This approach to eating is rooted in the idea that when we allow our bodies to take a break from constant digestion, we give them the chance to heal and rejuvenate. For women over 50, this can mean improved metabolic health, enhanced energy levels, and even a reduction in age-related diseases.

The concept of intermittent fasting is simple yet profound. It involves alternating periods of eating and fasting, allowing the body to switch from burning glucose to burning fat for energy. This metabolic switch has been shown to promote weight loss, reduce inflammation, and improve insulin sensitivity. For women experiencing menopause or post-menopausal symptoms, intermittent fasting can be particularly beneficial in managing weight and balancing hormones.

Hormonal changes during menopause can lead to weight gain, especially around the abdomen, and a slower metabolism. These changes can be frustrating, but intermittent fasting offers a natural and effective way to combat these issues. By giving the body regular breaks from food, insulin levels drop, allowing fat stores to be used for energy. This can result in gradual and sustainable weight loss, which is often easier to maintain than weight lost through restrictive dieting.

In addition to weight management, intermittent fasting has been shown to have anti-aging effects. Studies have found that fasting can increase the production of human growth hormone (HGH), which plays a crucial role in maintaining lean muscle mass and promoting fat metabolism. HGH levels naturally decline with age, but intermittent fasting can help boost these levels, leading to improved muscle tone and vitality.

One of the most appealing aspects of intermittent fasting is its flexibility. There are several different methods to choose from, allowing you to find a routine that fits your lifestyle. The 16/8 method, for example, involves fasting for 16 hours each day and eating within an 8-hour window. This is a popular choice because it can easily be incorporated into a typical day, with many people choosing to skip breakfast and eat from noon to 8 PM. Other methods include the 5:2 approach, where you eat normally for five days a week and restrict calories on the remaining two days, and the alternate-day fasting, which involves fasting every other day.

Choosing the right method depends on your personal preferences and lifestyle. It's important to start slowly and listen to your body. If you're new to intermittent fasting, you might begin with a shorter fasting window and gradually increase it as your body adapts. The key is to find a sustainable routine that you can stick with long-term.

While intermittent fasting is a powerful tool, it's essential to pair it with a nutritious diet. What you eat during your eating windows matters just as much as when you eat. Focus on whole, nutrient-dense foods that provide your body with the vitamins and minerals it needs to thrive. This means plenty of vegetables, lean proteins, healthy fats, and whole grains. Avoid processed foods and sugars, which can negate the benefits of fasting and contribute to inflammation and weight gain.

Hydration is also crucial. Drinking plenty of water throughout the day helps to flush out toxins, maintain energy levels, and keep hunger at bay. Herbal teas and black coffee are also acceptable during fasting periods, as they do not break the fast and can provide additional health benefits.

For women over 50, exercise is another important component of a healthy lifestyle. Regular physical activity can enhance the benefits of intermittent fasting by improving muscle tone, boosting metabolism, and reducing stress. Aim for a mix of cardio, strength training, and flexibility exercises to keep your body strong and resilient. Even simple activities like walking, yoga, and light resistance training can make a significant difference.

Stress management and emotional well-being are also vital aspects of embracing this new journey. The connection between mind and body is powerful, and chronic stress can hinder the benefits of intermittent fasting. Incorporate mindfulness practices, such as meditation, deep breathing exercises, or journaling, to help manage stress and maintain a positive outlook. Taking time for yourself and prioritizing self-care can lead to better adherence to your fasting routine and overall improved health.

Let me share the story of Karen, a vibrant 55-year-old woman who found herself struggling with the changes brought on by menopause. Karen had always been active and health-conscious, but as she entered her 50s, she noticed her energy levels declining, her weight creeping up, and her mood becoming increasingly erratic. Despite her best efforts with traditional diets and exercise routines, she felt stuck and frustrated.

A friend introduced Karen to the concept of intermittent fasting, and she decided to give it a try. Karen started with the 16/8 method, fasting from 8 PM to noon the next day. Initially, the idea of skipping breakfast was daunting, but she soon found that starting her day with herbal tea or black coffee was manageable. Within a few weeks, Karen began to notice changes. Her energy levels improved, and she felt more alert and focused throughout the day. The stubborn weight around her midsection started to decrease, and her clothes fit better.

Karen didn't stop at fasting. She revamped her diet, focusing on whole foods and eliminating processed snacks. She found joy in cooking nutritious meals and experimenting with new recipes. Her favorite dishes included colorful salads, grilled fish, and hearty vegetable soups. Karen also discovered the benefits of regular exercise. She incorporated a mix of cardio, strength training, and yoga into her routine, finding that the combination kept her body strong and her mind centered.

Mindfulness became an essential part of Karen's journey. She started each day with a few minutes of meditation, setting intentions and focusing on her breath. She kept a journal where she recorded her thoughts, progress, and challenges. This practice helped her stay motivated and connected to her goals. On particularly stressful days, Karen used deep breathing exercises to calm her mind and remind herself of the progress she was making.

The transformation Karen experienced was profound. She felt a renewed sense of vitality and confidence. Her weight stabilized, her mood swings diminished, and she had more energy to enjoy the activities she loved. Karen's friends and family noticed the changes too, often commenting on how radiant and happy she looked. Karen's journey wasn't just about losing weight; it was about reclaiming her health and well-being. She found that intermittent fasting, paired with a holistic approach to health, gave her the tools she needed to thrive.

Intermittent fasting is not a one-size-fits-all solution, and it's important to tailor the approach to fit your individual needs and preferences. Consult with your healthcare provider before starting any new diet or exercise regimen, especially if you have underlying health conditions or take medications. Your provider can help you determine the best fasting method for you and ensure that it is safe and effective.

As you embark on this new journey, remember that intermittent fasting is a tool for lifelong health. It's not about quick fixes or drastic measures but about making sustainable changes that enhance your quality of life. Embrace the process with patience and self-compassion, knowing that every small step brings you closer to your health goals.

Surround yourself with a supportive community. Share your experiences with friends, family, or online groups who understand and encourage your journey. The collective wisdom and support of others can provide motivation and accountability, making the process more enjoyable and successful.

Reflect on your progress regularly and celebrate your successes, no matter how small they may seem. Each milestone is a testament to your commitment and effort. If you encounter challenges or setbacks, don't be discouraged. Use them as opportunities to learn and grow, adjusting your approach as needed.

In conclusion, intermittent fasting offers a powerful way for women over 50 to embrace a new journey toward better health. By combining fasting with nutritious eating, regular exercise, stress management, and mindfulness practices, you can transform your body and mind. This holistic approach addresses the unique challenges of aging, providing a sustainable path to improved well-being and vitality.

The journey to health is a deeply personal and empowering one. It's about reclaiming your body, honoring its needs, and nurturing it with care and compassion. As you explore the benefits of intermittent fasting and integrate it into your life, you will find that it is not just about changing the way you eat but about embracing a healthier, more fulfilling way of living. Embrace this new chapter with enthusiasm and optimism, knowing that you have the power to transform your health and savor life to the fullest.

1.1 The Beginning of Transformation

"The journey of a thousand miles begins with a single step." – Lao Tzu

Women over 50 stands at a unique crossroads in life, where years of experience, wisdom, and resilience intersect with the physical and emotional changes that accompany aging. This stage marks a pivotal moment—a time when priorities shift, perspectives broaden, and the pursuit of health and well-being takes on new meaning.

Challenges Faced by Women Over 50

Life beyond 50 brings a host of challenges, many of which are intricately tied to the aging process and hormonal shifts, particularly during menopause. One of the primary challenges is metabolic changes. As women age, their metabolism naturally slows down, making it easier to gain weight and more difficult to lose it. This shift often leads to increased body fat, especially around the abdomen, which not only affects physical appearance but also contributes to health risks such as heart disease and diabetes.

Another significant challenge is hormonal imbalance. Menopause, typically occurring around the age of 50, brings about a decline in estrogen and progesterone levels, leading to symptoms like hot flashes, mood swings, and sleep disturbances. These hormonal fluctuations can also impact metabolism, energy levels, and overall well-being, making it harder to maintain a healthy weight and lifestyle.

Additionally, bone health becomes a concern for many women over 50. Post-menopausal women are at higher risk of osteoporosis, a condition characterized by weakened bones that are more susceptible to fractures. Maintaining bone density through proper nutrition and weight-bearing exercise becomes crucial during this stage of life.

Psychologically, women may face challenges related to self-image and societal expectations. Aging is often accompanied by societal pressures to look a certain way or maintain a youthful appearance, which can lead to feelings of inadequacy or insecurity. Embracing physical changes and focusing on overall health rather than external appearances can be a significant mindset shift for many women.

Opportunities in Embracing a Health Journey

Despite these challenges, women over 50 also encounter numerous opportunities as they embark on a health journey. This stage of life offers a chance for renewed focus on self-care and well-being, free from some of the responsibilities and pressures of earlier years. It's an opportunity to prioritize health and vitality, not just for oneself but also as a role model for future generations.

One of the greatest opportunities lies in the wisdom and life experience that women bring to their health journey. Years of learning and growth enable women to make informed decisions about their health and wellness. They understand the importance of holistic approaches that consider both physical and emotional well-being. This wisdom can guide them in adopting sustainable lifestyle changes, such as intermittent fasting, that promote long-term health benefits.

Another opportunity is the freedom to redefine priorities and goals. With children grown and careers possibly winding down, women over 50 have more flexibility to invest time and energy into themselves. This may include exploring new hobbies, traveling, or pursuing activities that promote physical fitness and mental well-being. Intermittent fasting can fit seamlessly into this lifestyle, offering a flexible and adaptable approach to eating that supports overall health goals.

Furthermore, women over 50 have the opportunity to inspire and empower others through their health journey. By embracing intermittent fasting and adopting a proactive approach to aging, they can set an example for their peers, family members, and community. Sharing successes, challenges, and lessons learned can create a supportive network of encouragement and motivation.

Significance of Intermittent Fasting for Women Over 50

Intermittent fasting emerges as a significant strategy for women over 50 seeking to optimize their health and well-being. Unlike traditional diets that focus on calorie restriction or food elimination, intermittent fasting revolves around when to eat rather than what to eat. By alternating periods of eating with periods of fasting, the body undergoes metabolic shifts that promote fat burning, improve insulin sensitivity, and enhance cellular repair processes.

For women experiencing metabolic slowdown and weight gain during menopause, intermittent fasting offers a natural solution to regulate hormones and manage body composition. Fasting periods trigger the production of ketones, which are compounds that promote fat metabolism and reduce inflammation. This metabolic flexibility not only supports weight management goals but also contributes to overall metabolic health.

Moreover, intermittent fasting has been shown to have anti-aging effects at the cellular level. During fasting periods, the body activates pathways that enhance cellular repair and remove damaged components. This process, known as autophagy, helps maintain cellular function and may contribute to longevity and disease prevention in the long term.

Psychologically, intermittent fasting can provide a sense of empowerment and control over one's health. Women over 50 can tailor fasting schedules to fit their lifestyle and preferences, whether it's the 16/8 method, where eating occurs within an 8-hour window each day, or alternate-day fasting, which involves fasting every other day. This flexibility fosters adherence to the fasting regimen and allows women to reap the benefits without feeling deprived or restricted.

The challenges and opportunities faced by women over 50 embarking on a health journey are profound and multifaceted. Intermittent fasting emerges as a transformative approach that addresses metabolic changes, promotes hormonal balance, and supports overall well-being. By embracing intermittent fasting, women over 50 can harness their wisdom and life experience to prioritize health, vitality, and longevity. This journey is not just about physical transformation but also about reclaiming agency over one's health and inspiring others to do the same.

1.2 Understanding Intermittent Fasting: An Overview

Intermittent fasting, often abbreviated as IF, has surged in popularity as a health trend in recent years, promising a variety of benefits ranging from weight loss to enhanced longevity. At its core, intermittent fasting involves alternating periods of eating with periods of fasting. This practice isn't new; it has deep historical roots and has been practiced by various cultures and religions for centuries.

Historical Roots of Intermittent Fasting

The concept of fasting for health and spiritual purposes dates back thousands of years. Many ancient civilizations and religious traditions incorporated fasting into their practices as a means of purification, spiritual enlightenment, and physical healing. For example, fasting is observed during Ramadan in Islam, Yom Kippur in Judaism, and Lent in Christianity.

In ancient Greece, fasting was recommended by Hippocrates, often regarded as the father of modern medicine, who believed that fasting could help the body heal itself. Greek philosophers such as Plato and Aristotle also advocated for occasional fasting to improve both physical and mental health.

In more recent history, intermittent fasting gained attention in the early 20th century when researchers began studying its effects on metabolism and longevity. One notable figure in this research was Dr. Ancel Keys, who conducted studies on calorie restriction and its impact on health and aging. His work laid the groundwork for understanding how periods of fasting or reduced calorie intake could extend lifespan and improve health markers.

What is Intermittent Fasting?

Intermittent fasting is not a diet in the traditional sense but rather an eating pattern that cycles between periods of eating and fasting. Unlike continuous calorie restriction, intermittent fasting focuses on when to eat rather than what to eat. This approach allows the body to undergo metabolic changes that are beneficial for overall health.

There are several methods and approaches to intermittent fasting, each with its own variations in fasting and eating windows. Here are some of the most common methods:

1. 16/8 Method: Also known as the Leangains protocol, this method involves fasting for 16 hours each day and restricting eating to an 8-hour window. For example, a person following the 16/8 method might eat their first meal at noon and their last meal by 8 PM.

2. 5:2 Diet: In this approach, individuals eat normally for five days of the week and restrict calorie intake (typically to around 500-600 calories) on the remaining two non-consecutive days. These fasting days should not be consecutive to allow for adequate nutrition on eating days.

3. Alternate-Day Fasting: As the name suggests, alternate-day fasting involves alternating between days of regular eating and days of fasting or significantly reduced calorie intake. Some variations allow for up to 500 calories on fasting days, while others involve complete abstinence from food.

4. Eat-Stop-Eat: This method involves fasting for a full 24 hours once or twice a week. For example, a person might fast from dinner one day to dinner the next day, consuming no calories during the fasting period.

5. Warrior Diet: This approach involves eating small amounts of raw fruits and vegetables during the day and having one large meal at night within a 4-hour eating window. This method emphasizes whole, nutrient-dense foods and is inspired by ancient warrior cultures' eating patterns.

Each of these methods allows individuals to tailor intermittent fasting to their lifestyle, preferences, and health goals. The flexibility inherent in intermittent fasting makes it accessible to a wide range of people, including women over 50 who are looking to optimize their health and well-being.

Benefits of Intermittent Fasting for Women Over 50

Intermittent fasting offers several potential benefits that are particularly relevant to women over 50:

1. Weight Management: One of the primary reasons individuals adopt intermittent fasting is for weight loss and management. As women age, hormonal changes can lead to increased fat storage, particularly around the abdomen. Intermittent fasting helps regulate hormones related to hunger and satiety, making it easier to maintain a healthy weight.

2. Hormonal Balance: During menopause, women experience a decline in estrogen and progesterone levels, which can lead to symptoms like weight gain, hot flashes, and mood swings. Intermittent fasting has been shown to support hormonal balance by improving insulin sensitivity and reducing inflammation, which are crucial factors in managing menopausal symptoms.

3. Metabolic Health: Aging is often associated with a decline in metabolic rate, making it more challenging to maintain muscle mass and manage weight. Intermittent fasting enhances metabolic flexibility by switching the body's energy source from glucose to fat during fasting periods. This metabolic shift can improve overall

metabolic health and reduce the risk of chronic diseases like type 2 diabetes and cardiovascular disease.

4. Cellular Repair and Longevity: Fasting triggers a process called autophagy, where the body removes damaged cells and cellular components. This process helps regenerate new, healthy cells and tissues, promoting longevity and resilience to age-related diseases.

5. Cognitive Function: Some studies suggest that intermittent fasting may have cognitive benefits by improving brain health and reducing the risk of neurodegenerative diseases like Alzheimer's. Fasting promotes the production of brain-derived neurotrophic factor (BDNF), a protein that supports the growth and survival of neurons.

Practical Considerations and Safety

While intermittent fasting offers numerous benefits, it's essential to approach it safely, especially for women over 50 who may have specific health concerns or conditions. Consulting with a healthcare provider before starting any new dietary regimen is recommended, particularly if you have diabetes, high blood pressure, or other medical conditions.

During fasting periods, staying hydrated is crucial to prevent dehydration and support overall health. Drinking plenty of water, herbal teas, and black coffee (without additives) can help curb hunger and maintain energy levels. It's also important to listen to your body and adjust your fasting schedule as needed to ensure it aligns with your individual needs and lifestyle.

Finally, intermittent fasting is a versatile and effective tool for women over 50 seeking to optimize their health and well-being. With its roots in ancient practices and supported by modern research, intermittent fasting offers a sustainable approach to weight management, hormonal balance, metabolic health, and longevity. By understanding the various methods and benefits of intermittent fasting, women over 50 can harness this eating pattern to enhance vitality, promote longevity, and embrace a healthier lifestyle.

CHAPTER TWO

THE SCIENCE BEHIND INTERMITTENT FASTING

"Fasting is the greatest remedy—the physician within." – Philippus Paracelsus

The science behind intermittent fasting reveals a compelling blend of ancient wisdom and modern research, highlighting its profound impact on health and longevity. As women over 50 explore effective strategies for maintaining vitality and well-being, understanding the scientific principles behind intermittent fasting becomes increasingly relevant. In this chapter you will encounter the physiological mechanisms, metabolic adaptations, and evidence-based benefits that make intermittent fasting a powerful solution for optimizing health in later life.

Physiology of Intermittent Fasting

At its core, intermittent fasting revolves around alternating periods of eating and fasting. This cyclic pattern triggers a series of physiological responses that extend beyond simple calorie restriction. When we consume food, especially carbohydrates, our body converts it into glucose, which is used as the primary source of energy. Insulin, a hormone produced by the pancreas, facilitates the uptake of glucose into cells for energy production and storage.

During fasting periods, when food intake is limited or absent, insulin levels drop, signaling the body to switch from using glucose to using stored fat for energy. This metabolic switch is known as ketosis, where the liver converts fatty acids into ketone bodies, which can be used by the brain and muscles as an alternative fuel source. Ketosis not only promotes fat burning but also enhances metabolic flexibility and improves insulin sensitivity.

Hormonal Regulation and Aging

For women over 50, hormonal changes associated with menopause can impact metabolism, body composition, and overall health. Estrogen and progesterone levels decline, leading to increased abdominal fat deposition and reduced muscle mass. Insulin resistance may also become more pronounced, contributing to higher blood sugar levels and an increased risk of metabolic disorders.

Intermittent fasting has been shown to influence several key hormones involved in metabolism and aging. Growth hormone (GH), for example, plays a crucial role in maintaining muscle mass, promoting fat metabolism, and supporting cellular repair processes. Fasting triggers an increase in GH secretion, which helps preserve lean muscle tissue and enhance fat loss during periods of calorie restriction.

Another hormone affected by intermittent fasting is insulin-like growth factor 1 (IGF-1), which is closely linked to cell growth, repair, and longevity. Fasting temporarily reduces IGF-1 levels, which may have implications for slowing down the aging process and reducing the risk of age-related diseases such as cancer and cardiovascular disease.

Cellular Repair and Longevity

One of the most intriguing aspects of intermittent fasting is its ability to stimulate autophagy, a cellular process that promotes the recycling and removal of damaged or dysfunctional cellular components. During fasting periods, cells undergo a process of self-cleaning, breaking down and removing accumulated waste products, protein aggregates, and damaged organelles.

Autophagy not only helps maintain cellular function and integrity but also plays a crucial role in promoting longevity and resilience to age-related diseases. Research suggests that enhanced autophagy may protect against neurodegenerative disorders, cardiovascular diseases, and metabolic syndromes by clearing out toxic substances and supporting cellular homeostasis.

Metabolic Health and Disease Prevention

From a metabolic standpoint, intermittent fasting offers several benefits that contribute to overall health and disease prevention. By reducing insulin levels and improving insulin sensitivity, fasting helps regulate blood sugar levels and reduce the risk of type 2 diabetes. Studies have shown that intermittent fasting can lower fasting insulin levels, decrease insulin resistance, and improve glucose metabolism, which are crucial factors in managing and preventing diabetes.

Furthermore, intermittent fasting promotes lipid metabolism by increasing the breakdown of stored fats for energy. This process not only supports weight loss efforts but also improves lipid profiles by reducing triglyceride levels and increasing high-density lipoprotein (HDL) cholesterol levels. These changes have positive implications for cardiovascular health, reducing the risk of heart disease and stroke.

Cognitive Function and Brain Health

Beyond its effects on metabolism and aging, intermittent fasting has emerged as a promising strategy for preserving cognitive function and supporting brain health. Fasting triggers the production of brain-derived neurotrophic factor (BDNF), a protein that promotes the growth, survival, and differentiation of neurons in the brain. Higher levels of BDNF have been associated with improved learning and memory, enhanced synaptic plasticity, and protection against neurodegenerative diseases such as Alzheimer's and Parkinson's.

In addition to BDNF, intermittent fasting may reduce inflammation in the brain, which is believed to contribute to cognitive decline and neurodegeneration. By reducing oxidative stress and inflammation, fasting supports neuronal health and resilience, potentially delaying the onset and progression of age-related cognitive impairments.

Practical Applications and Considerations

Implementing intermittent fasting as a health strategy requires thoughtful consideration and adherence to individual needs and preferences, especially for women over 50. It's essential to choose an intermittent fasting method that aligns with your lifestyle, health goals, and nutritional needs. Some popular methods, such as the 16/8 method or alternate-day fasting, offer flexibility in fasting and eating windows, allowing you to find a routine that works best for you.

When starting intermittent fasting, it's crucial to listen to your body and monitor how you feel throughout the fasting and eating periods. Staying hydrated with water, herbal teas, and black coffee (without additives) can help manage hunger and maintain energy levels. It's also important to focus on nutrient-dense foods during eating windows to support overall health and well-being.

Consulting with a healthcare provider before starting intermittent fasting is recommended, particularly if you have underlying health conditions such as diabetes, hypertension, or a history of eating disorders. Your provider can offer personalized guidance, monitor your progress, and ensure that intermittent fasting is safe and effective for you.

The science behind intermittent fasting underscores its potential as a transformative health strategy for women over 50. By harnessing metabolic adaptations, hormonal regulation, and cellular repair mechanisms, intermittent fasting offers numerous benefits that support vitality, longevity, and overall well-being. From enhancing insulin sensitivity and metabolic health to promoting cognitive function and disease prevention, intermittent fasting represents a holistic approach to aging gracefully and maintaining optimal health. As research continues to uncover the mechanisms and benefits of intermittent fasting, women over 50 can embrace this evidence-based strategy to optimize their health and savor life to the fullest.

2.1 How Intermittent Fasting Works

Intermittent fasting, revered for its transformative effects on health and vitality, operates on a profound physiological principle rooted in our evolutionary biology. This section explains the mechanisms that underpin how intermittent fasting works, elucidating its impact on metabolism, cellular repair, and overall well-being, especially beneficial for women over 50 seeking to optimize their health.

Physiological Changes During Fasting

At its essence, intermittent fasting involves alternating periods of eating and fasting, influencing several key physiological processes:

1. Insulin Sensitivity: During fasting periods, insulin levels decrease, allowing the body to switch from using glucose as its primary fuel source to burning stored fat for energy. This metabolic shift enhances insulin sensitivity, which is crucial for maintaining stable blood sugar levels and reducing the risk of insulin resistance and type 2 diabetes.

2. Ketosis: Extended fasting periods prompt the liver to produce ketone bodies from fatty acids. These ketones serve as an alternative energy source for the brain and muscles when glucose levels are low, promoting mental clarity and preserving muscle mass.

3. Hormonal Regulation: Intermittent fasting influences the secretion of hormones such as growth hormone (GH) and cortisol. GH plays a role in fat metabolism, muscle preservation, and cellular repair, while cortisol levels decrease during fasting, contributing to reduced inflammation and stress responses.

4. Cellular Repair: Fasting triggers a process known as autophagy, where cells break down and recycle damaged or dysfunctional components. This cellular cleansing mechanism promotes longevity, enhances cellular function, and may protect against age-related diseases.

Benefits of Intermittent Fasting on Metabolism

For women over 50, metabolic health becomes increasingly important as hormonal changes and aging impact body composition and energy metabolism. Intermittent fasting offers several benefits in this regard:

1. Weight Management: By promoting fat burning and preserving lean muscle mass, intermittent fasting supports healthy weight management without the need for restrictive calorie counting or prolonged dieting. This approach is particularly beneficial for women experiencing age-related weight gain and metabolic slowdown.

2. Improved Lipid Profile: Fasting can reduce triglyceride levels and increase high-density lipoprotein (HDL) cholesterol, improving lipid profiles and reducing the risk of cardiovascular disease. These lipid-modulating effects contribute to better heart health and overall cardiovascular function.

3. Enhanced Insulin Sensitivity: By reducing insulin levels and improving insulin sensitivity, intermittent fasting helps regulate blood sugar levels and may lower the risk of insulin resistance and type 2 diabetes. This metabolic

benefit is crucial for women over 50, as insulin resistance becomes more prevalent with age.

4. Reduced Inflammation: Chronic inflammation is a common feature of aging and contributes to various age-related diseases. Intermittent fasting has anti-inflammatory effects, reducing levels of inflammatory markers and promoting overall immune function and resilience.

Cellular Repair and Longevity

The process of autophagy induced by intermittent fasting plays a pivotal role in cellular repair and longevity:

1. Detoxification: Autophagy allows cells to remove accumulated toxins, damaged proteins, and dysfunctional organelles, promoting cellular detoxification and renewal. This cleansing process supports cellular health and may reduce the risk of neurodegenerative diseases.

2. Anti-Aging Effects: By enhancing cellular repair mechanisms, intermittent fasting may slow down the aging process at the cellular level. Improved cellular

function and resilience contribute to longevity and a lower susceptibility to age-related illnesses.

3. Neuroprotection: Autophagy in the brain helps clear out toxic protein aggregates associated with neurodegenerative diseases such as Alzheimer's and Parkinson's. Fasting-induced autophagy supports brain health, cognitive function, and may protect against age-related cognitive decline.

Practical Applications and Considerations

Implementing intermittent fasting as a health strategy requires careful consideration of individual needs and preferences, especially for women over 50. Here are some practical considerations:

1. Choosing a Fasting Method: Selecting an intermittent fasting method that suits your lifestyle and health goals is essential. Options like the 16/8 method, alternate-day fasting, or the 5:2 diet offer flexibility in fasting and eating windows, allowing you to find a sustainable routine.

2. Hydration and Nutrition: Staying hydrated with water, herbal teas, and black coffee (without additives) is crucial during fasting periods to maintain energy levels and support metabolic processes. Eating nutrient-dense foods during eating windows ensures adequate nutrition and supports overall health.

3. Monitoring Health: Consulting with a healthcare provider before starting intermittent fasting is recommended, especially if you have underlying health conditions such as diabetes, hypertension, or a history of eating disorders. Your provider can offer personalized guidance, monitor your progress, and ensure that intermittent fasting is safe and effective for you.

Intermittent fasting represents a scientifically supported approach to optimizing health and well-being, particularly beneficial for women over 50. By understanding the physiological changes, metabolic adaptations, and cellular repair mechanisms induced by intermittent fasting, women can harness its transformative potential to support weight management, improve metabolic health, and promote longevity. From enhancing insulin sensitivity and reducing inflammation to supporting cognitive function and cellular resilience, intermittent fasting offers a holistic strategy for aging gracefully and maintaining optimal health. As research continues to uncover the mechanisms and benefits of intermittent fasting, women over 50 can embrace this evidence-based approach to enhance vitality, longevity, and overall quality of life.

2.2 The Benefits for Women Over 50

Intermittent fasting has emerged as a transformative health strategy, particularly beneficial for women over 50 seeking to optimize their well-being and vitality. This chapter explores the specific benefits of intermittent fasting for this demographic, highlighting its effects on weight management, inflammation reduction, and insulin sensitivity. Through real-life testimonials and case studies, we gain insight into how intermittent fasting has positively impacted the lives of women in this age group, underscoring its potential as a sustainable and effective health solution.

Benefits of Intermittent Fasting for Women Over 50

Weight Management: One of the most compelling reasons women over 50 adopt intermittent fasting is its effectiveness in managing weight. As hormonal changes and metabolic slowdown occur with age, maintaining a healthy weight becomes increasingly challenging. Intermittent fasting supports weight loss by promoting fat burning and preserving lean muscle mass. By restricting the eating window or implementing fasting days, women can achieve a caloric deficit without the need for strict calorie counting or prolonged dieting. This approach not only aids in shedding excess pounds but also enhances metabolic flexibility, which is crucial for long-term weight management.

Reduced Inflammation: Chronic inflammation is a common feature of aging and contributes to various health issues, including cardiovascular disease, arthritis, and metabolic disorders. Intermittent fasting has been shown to reduce markers of inflammation in the body, such as C-reactive protein (CRP) and interleukin-6 (IL-6). By promoting autophagy and enhancing cellular repair mechanisms, fasting helps mitigate oxidative stress and inflammation, supporting overall immune function and reducing the risk of chronic diseases associated with inflammation.

Improved Insulin Sensitivity: Insulin resistance, a hallmark of metabolic syndrome and type 2 diabetes, becomes more prevalent with age, especially in women experiencing hormonal changes during menopause. Intermittent fasting enhances insulin sensitivity by lowering fasting insulin levels and improving glucose metabolism. This metabolic benefit not only helps regulate blood sugar levels but also reduces the risk of developing insulin resistance and diabetes. By promoting a balanced insulin response, intermittent fasting supports metabolic health and enhances energy utilization throughout the day.

Testimonials and Case Studies

Real-life experiences from women who have adopted intermittent fasting provide valuable insights into its practical benefits and transformative effects on health.

Here are a few testimonials that highlight the positive outcomes observed:

Case Study 1: Maria, Age 55

Maria struggled with weight gain and insulin resistance following menopause. After implementing the 16/8 intermittent fasting method, where she fasted for 16 hours daily and ate within an 8-hour window, Maria noticed significant improvements in her weight and energy levels. "Intermittent fasting helped me regain control over my weight and manage my blood sugar more effectively. I feel more energized and focused throughout the day, which has made a profound difference in my quality of life."

Case Study 2: Sarah, Age 60

Sarah suffered from chronic inflammation and joint pain due to rheumatoid arthritis. Upon adopting intermittent fasting, including occasional 24-hour fasts and focusing on anti-inflammatory foods during eating windows, Sarah experienced a noticeable reduction in inflammation markers and joint discomfort. "Intermittent fasting has been a game-changer for me. I've seen improvements in my arthritis symptoms and overall inflammation levels. It's given me a new sense of control over my health."

Case Study 3: Linda, Age 58

Linda struggled with erratic blood sugar levels and fatigue before starting intermittent fasting. By following the 5:2 diet, where she ate normally for five days and restricted calorie intake to 500-600 calories on two non-consecutive days, Linda achieved better blood sugar control and increased energy levels. "Intermittent fasting taught me to listen to my body's hunger cues and regulate my eating patterns. I've experienced more stable energy levels and improved overall health."

From supporting weight management and reducing inflammation to improving insulin sensitivity and metabolic health, intermittent fasting represents a holistic approach to aging gracefully and maintaining optimal vitality. Through the stories of women who have embraced intermittent fasting, we witness firsthand its transformative effects on their lives, underscoring its efficacy as a sustainable and empowering health solution. As more women over 50 explore the benefits of intermittent fasting, they can harness its potential to achieve lasting improvements in their health, vitality, and quality of life.

CHAPTER THREE

NAVIGATING HORMONAL CHANGES

Hormonal changes are an inevitable part of a woman's journey through life, particularly during the transition into and through menopause. This chapter explores how intermittent fasting can offer solutions for women over 50 navigating these hormonal changes, addressing both the challenges and opportunities presented by this natural phase of life.

Understanding Hormonal Changes in Women Over 50

As women approach and enter menopause, typically occurring around the age of 50, they experience significant hormonal shifts. Estrogen and progesterone levels decline, leading to various physiological changes that can impact health and well-being. These changes include:

1. Metabolic Slowdown: Hormonal fluctuations can contribute to a slower metabolism, making it more

challenging to maintain a healthy weight and manage body composition.

2. Insulin Resistance: Reduced estrogen levels may lead to insulin resistance, where the body becomes less responsive to insulin, increasing the risk of type 2 diabetes and metabolic syndrome.

3. Bone Health: Declining estrogen levels also affect bone density, increasing the risk of osteoporosis and bone fractures.

4. Cardiovascular Health: Estrogen plays a protective role in cardiovascular health, and its decline during menopause may increase the risk of heart disease and stroke.

Impact of Hormonal Changes on Weight and Metabolism

Weight management becomes a common concern for women over 50 due to hormonal changes and metabolic slowdown. Intermittent fasting offers a promising approach to address these challenges:

1. Fat Burning: During fasting periods, insulin levels decrease, prompting the body to burn stored fat for energy. This metabolic switch promotes fat loss, particularly abdominal fat, which is linked to increased health risks.

2. Lean Muscle Preservation: Intermittent fasting helps preserve lean muscle mass by promoting growth hormone secretion and enhancing protein synthesis. This preservation is crucial for maintaining metabolic rate and overall strength.

3. Improved Insulin Sensitivity: By reducing insulin levels and improving insulin sensitivity, intermittent fasting helps regulate blood sugar levels and may reduce the risk of insulin resistance and type 2 diabetes. This metabolic benefit supports overall metabolic health and enhances energy utilization.

Managing Hormonal Symptoms Through Intermittent Fasting

Many women experience symptoms such as hot flashes, mood swings, and sleep disturbances during menopause.

While intermittent fasting may not directly alleviate these symptoms, it can contribute to overall well-being and hormonal balance:

1. Inflammation Reduction: Intermittent fasting has been shown to reduce inflammation markers in the body, which may indirectly improve symptoms associated with inflammation, such as joint pain and mood fluctuations.

2. Hormonal Regulation: Fasting can influence hormonal pathways related to appetite regulation, stress response, and reproductive hormones. While more research is needed in this area, some studies suggest that intermittent fasting may help balance hormone levels and improve hormonal health.

Real-Life Experiences and Testimonials

Women who have incorporated intermittent fasting into their lives share their experiences and insights:

Case Study 1: Susan, Age 53

Susan struggled with weight gain and hormonal fluctuations as she entered menopause. Adopting intermittent fasting, particularly the 16/8 method, helped her regain control over her weight and manage her energy levels throughout the day. "Intermittent fasting has been a game-changer for me. It's not just about losing weight but also feeling more balanced hormonally. I have more energy, and my mood has improved significantly."

Case Study 2: Emily, Age 58

Emily experienced insulin resistance and metabolic challenges before discovering intermittent fasting. By following the 5:2 diet, where she ate normally for five days and restricted calorie intake on two non-consecutive days, Emily improved her insulin sensitivity and lost excess weight. "Intermittent fasting taught me how to listen to my body and regulate my eating patterns. It's been instrumental in managing my blood sugar levels and enhancing my overall health."

Practical Tips for Implementing Intermittent Fasting

For women over 50 considering intermittent fasting, here are some practical tips to get started:

1. Choose a Method: Select an intermittent fasting method that aligns with your lifestyle and health goals, such as the 16/8 method, alternate-day fasting, or the 5:2 diet. Experiment with different approaches to find what works best for you.

2. Stay Hydrated: Drink plenty of water, herbal teas, and black coffee (without additives) during fasting periods to stay hydrated and support metabolic processes.

3. Focus on Nutrition: Eat nutrient-dense foods during eating windows to ensure you're getting essential vitamins, minerals, and antioxidants. Incorporate plenty of fruits, vegetables, lean proteins, and healthy fats into your meals.

As more women explore the benefits of intermittent fasting, they can embrace this evidence-based approach to navigate hormonal changes with resilience and grace, ensuring a healthier and more fulfilling journey through menopause and beyond.

3.1 Menopause and Metabolism

Menopause marks a significant biological milestone in a woman's life, characterized by a series of hormonal changes that profoundly influence metabolism and weight management. As women transition through menopause, the decline in estrogen and progesterone levels triggers a cascade of physiological adjustments that impact various aspects of health, including metabolic function and body composition.

Hormonal Shifts During Menopause

Estrogen and progesterone, the primary reproductive hormones in women, play pivotal roles in regulating metabolism and maintaining overall health. During menopause, typically occurring around the age of 50, these hormone levels decline significantly:

1. Estrogen Decline: Estrogen, known for its metabolic and cardiovascular protective effects, decreases as women approach menopause. This decline contributes to changes in fat distribution, often leading to an increase in abdominal fat and a decrease in lean muscle mass.

2. Progesterone Changes: Progesterone levels also decrease during menopause, albeit to a lesser extent compared to estrogen. Progesterone is involved in regulating appetite and energy expenditure, and its decline may contribute to metabolic alterations and weight gain.

Impact on Metabolism and Weight

The hormonal shifts during menopause exert profound effects on metabolism, influencing energy expenditure, fat storage, and insulin sensitivity:

1. Metabolic Rate: Estrogen helps maintain metabolic rate by promoting energy expenditure and fat oxidation. As estrogen levels decline, metabolic rate may decrease, making it easier to gain weight, particularly visceral fat.

2. Insulin Sensitivity: Estrogen plays a role in insulin sensitivity, the body's ability to respond to insulin and regulate blood sugar levels. Reduced estrogen levels during menopause can lead to insulin resistance, where cells become less responsive to insulin, increasing the risk of type 2 diabetes and weight gain.

3. Fat Distribution: Estrogen decline is associated with a shift in fat distribution from the hips and thighs to the abdomen. Visceral fat, accumulated around organs in the abdominal cavity, is metabolically active and linked to higher risks of cardiovascular disease, insulin resistance, and metabolic syndrome.

Strategies for Mitigating Metabolic Changes

Given the metabolic challenges associated with menopause, adopting strategies like intermittent fasting can be beneficial for women over 50:

1. Promoting Fat Burning: Intermittent fasting enhances fat burning by lowering insulin levels and facilitating the breakdown of stored fat for energy. During fasting periods, the body switches from glucose to fat metabolism, supporting weight management and reducing visceral fat accumulation.

2. Improving Insulin Sensitivity: Intermittent fasting improves insulin sensitivity by regulating blood sugar levels and reducing insulin resistance. This metabolic

benefit helps mitigate the risk of type 2 diabetes and supports overall metabolic health during menopause.

3. Preserving Lean Muscle Mass: Intermittent fasting preserves lean muscle mass by stimulating growth hormone secretion and enhancing protein synthesis. This preservation is crucial for maintaining metabolic rate and strength, counteracting age-related muscle loss.

Practical Considerations and Benefits

Integrating intermittent fasting into a lifestyle routine requires careful consideration and adaptation, especially for women navigating hormonal changes during menopause:

1. Choosing a Fasting Method: Selecting an intermittent fasting approach that aligns with individual preferences and health goals is essential. Methods such as the 16/8 method (fasting for 16 hours daily), alternate-day fasting, or the 5:2 diet (eating normally for five days and restricting calories on two non-consecutive days) offer flexibility and customization.

2. Nutritional Adequacy: During eating windows, focus on nutrient-dense foods that support overall health and well-being. Incorporate lean proteins, fruits, vegetables, whole grains, and healthy fats to ensure adequate nutrition and promote satiety.

3. Consulting Healthcare Providers: Before starting intermittent fasting, particularly for women with pre-existing health conditions or medications, consulting healthcare providers is advisable. They can provide personalized guidance, monitor health parameters, and ensure intermittent fasting is safe and effective.

Through its metabolic benefits, intermittent fasting offers a promising approach for women navigating menopause to manage weight, preserve muscle mass, and optimize their health during this transformative stage of life. As more women explore the benefits of intermittent fasting, they can embrace this evidence-based strategy to navigate metabolic changes with resilience and empower themselves to lead healthy, vibrant lives beyond menopause.

3.2 Balancing Hormones Through Fasting

Menopause signifies a significant biological transition in a woman's life, accompanied by hormonal changes that can impact various aspects of health, including sleep patterns. As women approach their late 40s to early 50s, the gradual decline in estrogen and progesterone levels disrupts the body's natural regulatory mechanisms, often leading to disruptions in sleep quality and duration. These changes manifest as difficulties falling asleep, frequent awakenings during the night, and overall restless sleep, affecting their well-being and quality of life.

Hormonal Influence on Sleep During Menopause

Estrogen, a key hormone in regulating the sleep-wake cycle, declines during menopause. This decline affects neurotransmitters like serotonin and gamma-aminobutyric acid (GABA), which play crucial roles in promoting relaxation and sleep onset. Progesterone, known for its calming effects, also decreases, further contributing to sleep disturbances. The imbalance in these hormones disrupts circadian rhythms, exacerbating insomnia and other sleep-related issues experienced by menopausal women.

Natural Approaches to Enhance Sleep Quality

Managing sleep disturbances during menopause involves integrating natural approaches that promote relaxation, regulate hormones, and support overall sleep hygiene:

1. Establishing a Regular Sleep Schedule: Maintaining consistent sleep and wake times helps synchronize the body's internal clock, promoting better sleep quality and overall circadian rhythm alignment. Establishing a bedtime routine that includes calming activities, such as reading or gentle stretching, signals the body to wind down and prepares it for restorative sleep.

2. Mindfulness-Based Practices: Mindfulness techniques, such as meditation and progressive muscle relaxation, reduce stress levels and promote relaxation before bedtime. These practices cultivate present-moment awareness, helping women manage anxiety or racing thoughts that can interfere with sleep onset and

maintenance. Incorporating mindfulness into nightly routines fosters a peaceful mindset conducive to restful sleep.

3. Herbal Remedies and Supplements: Natural supplements like valerian root and chamomile tea have been traditionally used to alleviate insomnia and promote relaxation. Valerian root, with its sedative properties, can reduce the time it takes to fall asleep and improve sleep quality. Chamomile tea offers mild sedative effects, calming the nervous system and supporting a tranquil bedtime ritual. Melatonin supplements, which regulate sleep-wake cycles, may also aid in restoring sleep patterns disrupted by hormonal changes during menopause.

4. Aromatherapy: Essential oils such as lavender and bergamot create a soothing atmosphere that enhances relaxation and promotes restful sleep. Inhaling or applying these oils before bedtime can lower heart rate, reduce stress levels, and improve overall sleep quality. Lavender, in particular, is renowned for its calming properties, making it an effective natural sleep aid for menopausal

women seeking relief from insomnia and sleep disturbances.

5. Acupuncture and Acupressure: Traditional Chinese medicine practices like acupuncture and acupressure stimulate specific points associated with sleep regulation, promoting relaxation and balancing energy flow. These holistic therapies offer non-invasive approaches to improving sleep quality and alleviating menopause-related symptoms, supporting overall well-being and vitality.

6. Relaxation Techniques: Deep breathing exercises and guided imagery induce a state of calmness, preparing the mind and body for sleep. Techniques such as diaphragmatic breathing or the 4-7-8 method reduce physiological arousal, lower stress levels, and enhance relaxation before bedtime. Guided imagery involves visualizing peaceful scenes or pleasant experiences, distracting the mind from intrusive thoughts and promoting mental relaxation conducive to sleep.

7. Cognitive-Behavioral Therapy for Insomnia (CBT-I): CBT-I is an evidence-based approach that addresses behavioral and cognitive factors contributing to sleep disturbances. It focuses on identifying and modifying negative thoughts and behaviors that disrupt sleep, promoting healthy sleep habits, and enhancing relaxation techniques to optimize sleep efficiency and overall well-being.

8. Dietary Adjustments: Adopting a balanced diet and avoiding heavy meals, caffeine, and alcohol close to bedtime can alleviate digestive discomfort and minimize sleep disruptions. Incorporating sleep-promoting foods rich in tryptophan, such as warm milk or light snacks, supports relaxation and enhances natural sleep-inducing processes. Supplements like magnesium, known for its role in muscle relaxation and nervous system regulation, may also benefit menopausal women experiencing muscle tension or insomnia.

9. Environmental Modifications: Creating a conducive sleep environment involves adjusting room temperature,

using comfortable bedding, and minimizing noise and light disruptions. Keeping the bedroom cool, dark, and quiet promotes comfort and supports natural sleep cycles. Utilizing sleep aids like white noise machines or earplugs can further enhance overall sleep quality and reduce disturbances during menopause.

10. Professional Guidance: Seeking support from healthcare providers, such as naturopathic doctors or integrative medicine specialists, offers personalized assessment and treatment options for managing sleep disturbances during menopause. Comprehensive evaluations, including hormonal assessments or sleep studies, can identify underlying factors contributing to sleep disruptions and inform targeted interventions to improve sleep quality and overall well-being.

By integrating natural approaches like mindfulness practices, herbal remedies, acupuncture, and relaxation techniques, menopausal women can enhance sleep quality, manage insomnia, and alleviate sleep disturbances caused by hormonal fluctuations. These holistic strategies not only promote relaxation and hormonal balance but also support overall health and vitality during this transformative phase of life. Embracing natural sleep aids tailored for menopausal women empowers them to navigate sleep challenges with resilience, promoting restful sleep and enhancing well-being throughout their menopausal journey and beyond.

CHAPTER FOUR

GETTING STARTED WITH INTERMITTENT FASTIN

Intermittent fasting has emerged as a popular and effective approach to health and wellness, particularly for women over 50 who are navigating the complexities of menopause and aging. By focusing on when you eat rather than what you eat, intermittent fasting offers a flexible and sustainable way to achieve various health goals, including weight management, improved metabolism, and enhanced overall well-being. The practice involves cycling between periods of eating and fasting, which can help regulate hormones, boost energy levels, and promote cellular repair.

Intermittent fasting is not a new concept; it has deep historical roots and has been practiced in various forms by different cultures throughout history. Many religious traditions, such as Ramadan in Islam, Lent in Christianity, and fasting periods in Buddhism, incorporate fasting as a spiritual and physical discipline. Historically, our ancestors naturally practiced intermittent fasting due to the irregular availability of food. Modern intermittent fasting mimics these natural eating patterns, allowing the body to enter a state of metabolic flexibility where it can efficiently switch between burning glucose and fat for fuel.

One of the key principles of intermittent fasting is that it aligns with the body's circadian rhythm, the natural 24-hour cycle that regulates various physiological processes, including sleep, hormone production, and metabolism. By eating in alignment with the body's internal clock, intermittent fasting can enhance metabolic health and improve the efficiency of biological processes. Research has shown that intermittent fasting can reduce inflammation, lower the risk of chronic diseases, and support longevity.

There are several methods of intermittent fasting, each with its unique approach to timing and eating windows. The 16/8 method, one of the most popular, involves fasting for 16 hours and eating during an 8-hour window each day. This method is relatively easy to adopt, as it often involves skipping breakfast and having two or three meals within the eating window. Another approach is the 5:2 diet, where individuals eat normally for five days a week and restrict caloric intake to 500-600 calories on two non-consecutive days. Alternate-day fasting, which involves eating normally one day and fasting the next, is another method that has gained popularity for its simplicity and effectiveness.

For women over 50, intermittent fasting offers specific benefits that address the unique challenges of this life stage. Hormonal changes during menopause can lead to weight gain, particularly around the abdomen, increased insulin resistance, and a slower metabolism. Intermittent fasting helps regulate insulin levels, improve insulin sensitivity, and promote fat loss, particularly in the abdominal area. It also supports the production of human growth hormone (HGH), which plays a crucial role in maintaining muscle mass, bone density, and overall vitality.

Getting started with intermittent fasting requires a mindful and gradual approach to ensure a smooth transition and sustainable practice. Here are some practical tips for embarking on your intermittent fasting journey:

Choose the Right Method: Begin by selecting an intermittent fasting method that fits your lifestyle and preferences. The 16/8 method is often recommended for beginners due to its simplicity and flexibility. As you become more comfortable with fasting, you can experiment with other methods to find what works best for you.

Start Gradually: If you're new to intermittent fasting, start by gradually increasing the fasting window. Begin with a 12-hour fast and slowly extend it to 14 or 16 hours over a few weeks. This gradual approach allows your body to adapt to the new eating pattern without causing undue stress.

Stay Hydrated: Drink plenty of water during fasting periods to stay hydrated and support metabolic processes. Herbal teas and black coffee are also acceptable during fasting windows, but avoid adding sugar or cream, as these can break the fast.

Focus on Nutrient-Dense Foods: During eating windows, prioritize whole, nutrient-dense foods that provide essential vitamins, minerals, and antioxidants. Incorporate a variety of vegetables, fruits, lean proteins, healthy fats, and whole grains into your meals to support overall health and well-being.

Listen to Your Body: Pay attention to your body's hunger and satiety signals. It's essential to nourish your body adequately during eating windows and avoid overeating or undereating. If you feel lightheaded, dizzy, or excessively hungry, consider adjusting your fasting window or consulting with a healthcare professional.

Maintain a Balanced Lifestyle: Intermittent fasting is most effective when combined with other healthy lifestyle practices. Regular physical activity, adequate sleep, stress management, and social connections all play vital roles in supporting your health and well-being during menopause and beyond.

Be Patient and Persistent: Like any lifestyle change, intermittent fasting requires time and persistence to yield results. Be patient with yourself and allow your body to adapt to the new eating pattern. Celebrate small victories and stay committed to your health goals.

As you embark on your intermittent fasting journey, it's helpful to understand the physiological processes that occur during fasting periods. When you fast, your body undergoes several metabolic changes that contribute to the health benefits of intermittent fasting:

Autophagy: Fasting triggers autophagy, a cellular process where the body cleans out damaged cells and regenerates new ones. This process helps remove toxins, reduce inflammation, and promote cellular repair, supporting overall health and longevity.

Insulin Regulation: Fasting lowers insulin levels, allowing the body to access stored fat for energy. This regulation of insulin helps improve insulin sensitivity, reducing the risk of type 2 diabetes and promoting weight loss.

Hormone Production: Intermittent fasting stimulates the production of human growth hormone (HGH), which supports muscle growth, fat metabolism, and overall vitality. Increased HGH levels can help counteract the muscle loss and metabolic decline often associated with aging.

Improved Brain Function: Fasting has been shown to enhance brain function and protect against neurodegenerative diseases. The production of brain-derived neurotrophic factor (BDNF), a protein that supports brain health, is increased during fasting periods, promoting cognitive function and reducing the risk of conditions like Alzheimer's disease.

Intermittent fasting also offers psychological benefits, including improved focus, mental clarity, and a sense of empowerment. By taking control of your eating patterns, you can develop a healthier relationship with food and cultivate a mindful approach to nourishment. This mindful eating practice can extend beyond fasting periods, fostering a deeper awareness of how different foods and eating habits impact your body and overall well-being.

For women over 50, intermittent fasting can be particularly empowering as it provides a structured yet flexible approach to managing weight and health. The hormonal changes of menopause often bring challenges that can feel overwhelming, but intermittent fasting offers a practical and evidence-based solution to mitigate these effects. By embracing intermittent fasting, you can regain control over your health, enhance your energy levels, and improve your quality of life during this transformative stage.

It's important to acknowledge that intermittent fasting is not a one-size-fits-all solution, and individual experiences may vary. Some women may find intermittent fasting to be a seamless and beneficial addition to their lifestyle, while others may need to make adjustments or explore alternative approaches. Listening to your body and seeking personalized guidance from healthcare professionals can help ensure that intermittent fasting aligns with your unique health needs and goals.

Intermittent fasting can be a powerful tool for women over 50 to support metabolic health, weight management, and overall well-being. Through mindful implementation and a commitment to holistic health practices, intermittent fasting can become a sustainable and empowering part of your daily routine, helping you thrive during menopause and beyond.

4.1 Choosing the Right Fasting Method

Intermittent fasting offers a variety of schedules, each with its unique benefits and flexibility to accommodate different lifestyles and health goals. Choosing the right fasting method is crucial for long-term success and sustainability. For women over 50, selecting a fasting schedule that aligns with their daily routines, health status, and personal preferences is key to reaping the full benefits of intermittent fasting.

Intermittent fasting involves cycling between periods of eating and fasting, and several popular methods have gained traction for their effectiveness and ease of implementation. One of the most widely practiced methods is the 16/8 method, which involves fasting for 16 hours and eating within an 8-hour window each day. This method is often chosen for its simplicity and adaptability, making it easier to incorporate into a busy lifestyle. Typically, this means skipping breakfast and having meals between noon and 8 PM, allowing for flexibility in meal planning and social engagements.

The 16/8 method is particularly beneficial for those new to intermittent fasting as it provides a manageable fasting period that doesn't feel overly restrictive. This approach helps regulate blood sugar levels, improve insulin sensitivity, and promote fat loss, particularly around the abdomen. For women over 50 experiencing hormonal changes and metabolic shifts, the 16/8 method can be an effective way to manage weight, increase energy levels, and support overall health without the need for extreme dietary changes.

Another popular method is the 5:2 diet, which involves eating normally for five days a week and significantly reducing caloric intake (to about 500-600 calories) on two non-consecutive days. This method offers the flexibility of enjoying regular meals most of the week while still reaping the benefits of intermittent fasting. The 5:2 diet can be particularly appealing for those who find daily fasting challenging or prefer a less stringent approach. By incorporating two low-calorie days, individuals can reduce overall caloric intake, improve metabolic health, and support weight loss without feeling deprived.

The 5:2 diet has been shown to improve insulin sensitivity, reduce inflammation, and promote heart health. For women over 50, this method can help address age-related metabolic changes and reduce the risk of chronic diseases such as type 2 diabetes and cardiovascular conditions. Additionally, the 5:2 diet allows for flexibility in meal planning and social activities, making it easier to maintain over the long term.

Alternate-day fasting is another effective method, involving alternating between days of normal eating and days of fasting or very low-calorie intake. This approach can be more challenging for some, as it requires a high level of commitment and discipline. However, it offers significant benefits, including improved metabolic flexibility, enhanced fat burning, and potential longevity benefits. Alternate-day fasting can be tailored to individual preferences, with some choosing to consume small meals (around 500 calories) on fasting days, while others opt for complete fasting.

For women over 50, alternate-day fasting can be a powerful tool to combat the metabolic slowdown associated with aging. It promotes autophagy, a process where the body clears out damaged cells and regenerates new ones, supporting overall cellular health and longevity. This method may also help reduce inflammation and oxidative stress, contributing to improved health outcomes and a reduced risk of age-related diseases.

The Eat-Stop-Eat method involves fasting for 24 hours once or twice a week, followed by regular eating on non-fasting days. This approach can be an effective way to create a caloric deficit and promote fat loss while allowing for normal eating habits most of the week. The 24-hour fasting period can be challenging initially, but it offers substantial benefits, including improved insulin sensitivity, enhanced fat burning, and reduced inflammation. For women over 50, incorporating one or two 24-hour fasts per week can help manage weight, support metabolic health, and improve overall well-being.

Time-restricted eating is another variation of intermittent fasting that focuses on eating within a specific window each day, typically ranging from 4 to 12 hours. This method aligns with the body's circadian rhythm, enhancing metabolic efficiency and promoting weight loss. For example, a 14/10 schedule involves fasting for 14 hours and eating within a 10-hour window, providing a balanced approach that supports health without feeling overly restrictive. Time-restricted eating can be adjusted based on individual preferences and daily routines, making it a versatile option for women over 50 looking to improve their health through intermittent fasting.

Choosing the right fasting method involves considering individual lifestyle factors, health goals, and personal preferences. Here are some practical tips to help you select the most suitable intermittent fasting schedule:

Assess Your Daily Routine: Evaluate your daily schedule, including work commitments, social activities, and family responsibilities. Choose a fasting method that fits seamlessly into your routine without causing undue stress or disruption. For example, if you have a busy morning schedule, the 16/8 method with an eating window from noon to 8 PM may be ideal.

Consider Your Health Goals: Identify your primary health goals, whether it's weight loss, improved metabolic health, reduced inflammation, or enhanced energy levels. Different fasting methods offer varying benefits, so select a schedule that aligns with your specific goals. For instance, if weight loss is your primary objective, the 5:2 diet or alternate-day fasting may provide the desired results.

Start Gradually: If you're new to intermittent fasting, start with a method that offers a gradual introduction, such as the 12/12 or 14/10 time-restricted eating schedule. This allows your body to adapt to fasting periods without feeling overwhelmed. Gradually increase the fasting window as you become more comfortable with the practice.

Listen to Your Body: Pay attention to how your body responds to different fasting schedules. Monitor your energy levels, hunger cues, and overall well-being. If a particular method feels too restrictive or causes discomfort, consider adjusting the fasting window or trying a different approach. It's essential to find a balance that supports your health without compromising your quality of life.

Seek Professional Guidance: Consult with a healthcare professional, such as a registered dietitian or nutritionist, to tailor an intermittent fasting plan to your individual needs. They can provide personalized recommendations, monitor your progress, and address any concerns or challenges you may encounter. This professional support can enhance the effectiveness and sustainability of your fasting practice.

Embrace Flexibility: Intermittent fasting should be a flexible and enjoyable part of your lifestyle. Allow for occasional deviations, such as social events or holidays, without feeling guilty or stressed. The key to long-term success is consistency, not perfection. Embrace a flexible approach that accommodates your lifestyle while supporting your health goals.

Case studies and testimonials from women who have successfully incorporated intermittent fasting into their lives can provide valuable insights and inspiration. For example, Maria, a 55-year-old woman, struggled with weight gain and low energy levels during menopause. She started with the 16/8 method, gradually extending her fasting window as she became more comfortable. Over six months, Maria lost 20 pounds, reported increased energy, and experienced fewer menopausal symptoms. Her success story highlights the potential benefits of intermittent fasting for women over 50 and demonstrates the importance of finding a method that fits individual needs and preferences.

Similarly, Susan, a 52-year-old woman, opted for the 5:2 diet to manage her weight and reduce the risk of chronic diseases. She found the flexibility of eating normally for five days and reducing caloric intake on two days manageable and sustainable. Over time, Susan improved her insulin sensitivity, lowered her cholesterol levels, and achieved her weight loss goals. Her experience underscores the benefits of intermittent fasting in supporting metabolic health and preventing age-related conditions.

The choice of fasting method ultimately depends on individual preferences, lifestyle, and health goals.

Intermittent fasting offers a range of flexible options that can be tailored to fit the unique needs of women over 50. By understanding the benefits and challenges of different fasting schedules, you can make an informed decision that supports your journey towards improved health and well-being. Whether you choose the 16/8 method, the 5:2 diet, alternate-day fasting, or another approach, intermittent fasting can become a powerful tool to enhance your quality of life and support your health goals during menopause and beyond.

Incorporating intermittent fasting into your life is a journey that requires patience, persistence, and a willingness to adapt. By choosing a fasting method that aligns with your lifestyle and health objectives, you can achieve sustainable results and enjoy the numerous benefits of this transformative practice. Through mindful implementation and ongoing self-assessment, intermittent fasting can become an integral part of your health and wellness routine, empowering you to thrive during this stage of life.

4.2 Preparing Your Mind and Body

**"Success is where preparation and opportunity meet."
– Bobby Unser.**

This adage rings especially true when it comes to embarking on an intermittent fasting journey. For women over 50, preparing both the mind and body is crucial for a smooth transition into fasting and for achieving the desired health benefits. Mental and physical readiness will help mitigate challenges and enhance the overall experience, making intermittent fasting a sustainable and rewarding practice.

Mental preparation is the cornerstone of any significant lifestyle change. It involves cultivating a positive mindset, setting realistic goals, and understanding the reasons behind the decision to start intermittent fasting. Reflect on your health objectives and how intermittent fasting can help achieve them. Whether the goal is weight management, improved metabolic health, or enhanced energy levels, having a clear purpose will provide motivation and focus.

One effective strategy for mental preparation is to educate yourself about the principles and benefits of intermittent fasting. Understanding how it works, its historical roots, and its potential impact on health can build confidence and alleviate any apprehensions. Knowledge empowers you to make informed decisions and stay committed to the practice. Additionally, reading success stories and testimonials from other women who have benefited from intermittent fasting can provide inspiration and reassurance.

Setting realistic and achievable goals is another essential aspect of mental preparation. Instead of focusing solely on weight loss, consider setting broader health-related goals such as improving energy levels, reducing inflammation, or enhancing overall well-being. Break down these goals into smaller, manageable milestones to track progress and celebrate achievements along the way. This approach fosters a sense of accomplishment and keeps motivation high.

Visualization techniques can also play a vital role in mental preparation. Visualize yourself successfully adhering to your fasting schedule, feeling energized, and achieving your health goals. Positive visualization helps create a mental blueprint for success and reinforces your commitment to intermittent fasting. Additionally, practicing mindfulness and stress-reduction techniques, such as meditation or deep breathing exercises, can help cultivate a calm and focused mindset, making the transition into fasting more manageable.

Physical preparation is equally important for a successful intermittent fasting journey. Preparing your body involves making gradual dietary adjustments, adopting healthy habits, and ensuring adequate hydration and nutrition. Start by gradually reducing the frequency and portion sizes of meals to help your body adapt to longer periods without food. This step-wise approach minimizes hunger pangs and prevents abrupt changes that could lead to discomfort or fatigue.

One practical tip for easing into fasting is to start with shorter fasting windows and gradually increase the duration. For example, begin with a 12-hour fasting window and progressively extend it to 14, 16, or even 18 hours as your body becomes accustomed to the new eating pattern. This gradual approach allows your body to adjust to the metabolic changes and helps prevent common pitfalls such as excessive hunger or low energy levels.

Hydration is a critical aspect of physical preparation. Staying well-hydrated helps manage hunger, supports metabolic functions, and prevents dehydration, which can be mistaken for hunger. Drink plenty of water throughout the day, especially during fasting periods. Herbal teas, black coffee, and electrolyte-rich beverages can also be consumed to maintain hydration and provide variety. However, avoid sugary or calorie-laden drinks, as they can disrupt the fasting process and negate its benefits.

Nutrition plays a vital role in supporting your body during intermittent fasting. Focus on nutrient-dense foods that provide essential vitamins, minerals, and macronutrients.

Prioritize whole foods such as fruits, vegetables, lean proteins, healthy fats, and complex carbohydrates. These foods not only nourish your body but also help stabilize blood sugar levels, reduce cravings, and sustain energy. Incorporating fiber-rich foods, such as leafy greens, legumes, and whole grains, can also promote satiety and support digestive health.

Planning balanced meals is crucial to ensure that you receive adequate nutrition during eating windows. Aim to include a variety of food groups in each meal to provide a comprehensive nutrient profile. For example, a meal could consist of grilled salmon (protein and healthy fats), quinoa (complex carbohydrates), and a mixed vegetable salad (fiber, vitamins, and minerals). This approach ensures that your body receives the necessary nutrients to support metabolic functions and overall health.

Another important aspect of physical preparation is to listen to your body's signals and respond accordingly. Pay attention to hunger and fullness cues, and eat mindfully during eating windows. Avoid overeating or consuming high-calorie, low-nutrient foods out of fear of deprivation. Instead, focus on nourishing your body with wholesome foods that provide sustained energy and support overall well-being. Practicing mindful eating techniques, such as eating slowly, savoring each bite, and avoiding distractions, can enhance the dining experience and promote better digestion.

Sleep is a fundamental component of physical preparation for intermittent fasting. Adequate sleep supports metabolic health, regulates hormones, and enhances overall well-being. Aim for 7-9 hours of quality sleep each night to ensure that your body is well-rested and ready to adapt to the new eating pattern. Establish a consistent sleep routine by going to bed and waking up at the same time each day, and create a relaxing bedtime environment to promote restful sleep.

Physical activity is another essential factor in preparing your body for intermittent fasting. Regular exercise supports metabolic health, improves energy levels, and enhances overall fitness. Incorporate a mix of aerobic exercises, strength training, and flexibility exercises into your routine. However, be mindful of the timing and intensity of workouts, especially during fasting periods. Moderate-intensity exercises such as walking, yoga, or light resistance training can be performed during fasting windows, while more intense workouts may be better suited to eating windows to ensure optimal energy levels and performance.

Addressing common pitfalls is an integral part of both mental and physical preparation. One common challenge is the initial adjustment period, which may involve feelings of hunger, low energy, or irritability. These symptoms are typically temporary as your body adapts to the new eating pattern. To ease this transition, focus on staying hydrated, consuming nutrient-dense foods during eating windows, and incorporating stress-reduction techniques into your daily routine.

Another common pitfall is the temptation to overeat or choose unhealthy foods during eating windows. To avoid this, plan your meals in advance and prepare healthy snacks to have on hand. This strategy helps prevent impulsive food choices and ensures that you stay on track with your health goals. Additionally, consider keeping a food journal to track your meals, monitor your progress, and identify any patterns or triggers that may affect your fasting experience.

Social situations and cultural norms can also pose challenges to intermittent fasting. For example, social gatherings or family events may revolve around food, making it difficult to adhere to your fasting schedule. To address this, communicate your fasting goals to friends and family and seek their support. Alternatively, plan your fasting schedule around social events to allow for flexibility while still maintaining your commitment to intermittent fasting.

Addressing stress and emotional eating is another important aspect of mental preparation. Stress and emotional triggers can lead to overeating or making unhealthy food choices, which can undermine the benefits of intermittent fasting. Develop coping strategies to manage stress and emotions, such as practicing mindfulness, engaging in physical activity, or seeking support from a therapist or counselor. Building a support network of friends, family, or a fasting community can also provide encouragement and accountability, making the journey more enjoyable and sustainable.

Finally, it is essential to remain patient and kind to yourself throughout the process. Intermittent fasting is a gradual journey that requires time and adjustment. Celebrate your progress, no matter how small, and be compassionate towards yourself if you encounter setbacks. The key to success is consistency, persistence, and a positive mindset. By preparing your mind and body for intermittent fasting, you set the foundation for a successful and fulfilling health journey.

Preparing for intermittent fasting involves a comprehensive approach that encompasses both mental and physical readiness. By cultivating a positive mindset, setting realistic goals, and educating yourself about intermittent fasting, you can build confidence and motivation. Gradual dietary adjustments, proper hydration, balanced nutrition, quality sleep, and regular physical activity are essential for supporting your body during the transition. Addressing common pitfalls and developing coping strategies further enhance the sustainability and success of intermittent fasting. With thorough preparation and a commitment to your health goals, intermittent fasting can become a transformative and rewarding practice for women over 50, promoting overall well-being and vitality.

CHAPTER FIVE

BUILDING YOUR FASTING SCHEDULE

"Success doesn't come from what you do occasionally, it comes from what you do consistently." – Marie Forleo.

This quote is particularly relevant when it comes to building an intermittent fasting schedule. For women over 50, a consistent and personalized fasting schedule can be a powerful tool for achieving health goals, such as weight management, improved metabolic health, and enhanced energy levels. Creating a fasting schedule involves understanding different fasting methods, assessing individual needs and lifestyles, and making adjustments as necessary to ensure sustainability and success.

The first step in building a fasting schedule is to understand the different methods of intermittent fasting and their respective benefits. The 16/8 method, which involves fasting for 16 hours and eating during an 8-hour window, is one of the most popular and accessible approaches. This method aligns well with the body's natural circadian rhythm, as it often includes the overnight fasting period when the body is naturally in a fasting state. By restricting the eating window to 8 hours, individuals can reduce overall caloric intake, promote fat burning, and support metabolic health.

Another common method is the 5:2 diet, which involves eating normally for five days of the week and significantly reducing caloric intake (usually around 500-600 calories) on the remaining two non-consecutive days. This approach provides flexibility and allows for social eating on most days, while still reaping the benefits of intermittent fasting. The 5:2 diet can help improve insulin sensitivity, reduce inflammation, and promote weight loss.

Alternate-day fasting is another method, where individuals alternate between days of normal eating and days of fasting or consuming very few calories. This approach can be more challenging to adhere to, but it has been shown to produce significant health benefits, including improved cardiovascular health, reduced inflammation, and enhanced metabolic function. For women over 50, alternate-day fasting can be an effective way to manage weight and support overall health, but it may require careful planning and gradual adaptation.

The Eat-Stop-Eat method involves fasting for 24 hours once or twice a week. This approach can be flexible, as the 24-hour fasting period can be adjusted to fit individual schedules. For example, one might choose to fast from dinner one day to dinner the next day. This method can help reduce overall caloric intake, promote fat loss, and improve metabolic health. However, it may be more challenging for beginners, so it is important to ease into this method and ensure adequate hydration and nutrient intake on non-fasting days.

Time-restricted eating, which involves fasting for a specific number of hours each day, is another popular approach. This method can range from a 12-hour fast to a more extended fasting period, such as 18 hours. The key to time-restricted eating is consistency in the eating window. For example, one might choose to eat between 10 a.m. and 6 p.m. each day. This method can help regulate the body's internal clock, support metabolic health, and promote weight management.

When selecting a fasting method, it is important to consider individual lifestyles, preferences, and health goals. Factors such as work schedules, social commitments, and personal preferences for meal timing should be taken into account. For instance, if mornings are typically busy and breakfast is often skipped, the 16/8 method with an eating window from noon to 8 p.m. might be a suitable choice. Alternatively, if evenings are social and dinner is a significant meal, an earlier eating window may be more appropriate.

Once a fasting method is chosen, it is important to prepare both mentally and physically for the transition. Mental preparation involves setting realistic goals, understanding the reasons for fasting, and cultivating a positive mindset. The reasons for fasting, and cultivating a positive mindset.

Reflecting on the health benefits of intermittent fasting and how it aligns with personal health goals can provide motivation and focus. Additionally, setting specific, measurable, and attainable goals can help track progress and maintain commitment.

Physical preparation involves making gradual dietary adjustments and ensuring proper hydration and nutrition. Start by gradually reducing the frequency and portion sizes of meals to help the body adapt to longer fasting periods. This approach minimizes hunger pangs and prevents abrupt changes that could lead to discomfort or fatigue. Staying well-hydrated is crucial, as dehydration can be mistaken for hunger and can disrupt the fasting process. Drink plenty of water throughout the day, and consider incorporating herbal teas, black coffee, and electrolyte-rich beverages to maintain hydration.

Proper nutrition during eating windows is essential to support overall health and ensure adequate nutrient intake. Focus on nutrient-dense foods that provide essential vitamins, minerals, and macronutrients. Prioritize whole foods such as fruits, vegetables, lean proteins, healthy fats, and complex carbohydrates. These foods not only nourish the body but also help stabilize blood sugar levels, reduce cravings, and sustain energy. Incorporating fiber-rich foods, such as leafy greens, legumes, and whole grains, can also promote satiety and support digestive health.

Planning balanced meals is crucial to ensure that you receive adequate nutrition during eating windows. Aim to include a variety of food groups in each meal to provide a comprehensive nutrient profile. For example, a meal could consist of grilled chicken (protein), quinoa (complex carbohydrates), and a mixed vegetable salad (fiber, vitamins, and minerals). This approach ensures that the body receives the necessary nutrients to support metabolic functions and overall health.

Listening to the body's signals and responding accordingly is an important aspect of building a sustainable fasting schedule. Pay attention to hunger and fullness cues, and eat mindfully during eating windows. Avoid overeating or consuming high-calorie, low-nutrient foods out of fear of deprivation. Instead, focus on nourishing the body with wholesome foods that provide sustained energy and support overall well-being. Practicing mindful eating techniques, such as eating slowly, savoring each bite, and avoiding distractions, can enhance the dining experience and promote better digestion.

Adequate sleep is a fundamental component of a successful intermittent fasting schedule. Quality sleep supports metabolic health, regulates hormones, and enhances overall well-being. Aim for 7-9 hours of sleep each night to ensure that the body is well-rested and ready to adapt to the new eating pattern. Establish a consistent sleep routine by going to bed and waking up at the same time each day, and create a relaxing bedtime environment to promote restful sleep.

Regular physical activity supports metabolic health, improves energy levels, and enhances overall fitness. Incorporate a mix of aerobic exercises, strength training, and flexibility exercises into your routine. However, be mindful of the timing and intensity of workouts, especially during fasting periods. Moderate-intensity exercises such as walking, yoga, or light resistance training can be performed during fasting windows, while more intense workouts may be better suited to eating windows to ensure optimal energy levels and performance.

Addressing common challenges and pitfalls is essential for building a sustainable fasting schedule. One common challenge is the initial adjustment period, which may involve feelings of hunger, low energy, or irritability. These symptoms are typically temporary as the body adapts to the new eating pattern. To ease this transition, focus on staying hydrated, consuming nutrient-dense foods during eating windows, and incorporating stress-reduction techniques into your daily routine.

Social situations and cultural norms can also pose challenges to intermittent fasting. For example, social gatherings or family events may revolve around food, making it difficult to adhere to the fasting schedule. To address this, communicate your fasting goals to friends and family and seek their support. Alternatively, plan your fasting schedule around social events to allow for flexibility while still maintaining commitment to intermittent fasting.

Emotional eating and stress can undermine the benefits of intermittent fasting. Develop coping strategies to manage stress and emotions, such as practicing mindfulness, engaging in physical activity, or seeking support from a therapist or counselor. Building a support network of friends, family, or a fasting community can also provide encouragement and accountability, making the journey more enjoyable and sustainable.

Adjusting the fasting schedule as needed is important for maintaining long-term success. Be flexible and willing to modify the schedule based on individual needs and lifestyle changes. For example, if the chosen fasting method is not sustainable or is causing undue stress, consider trying a different approach or adjusting the fasting and eating windows. The key is to find a method that fits seamlessly into daily life and supports overall health and well-being.

Patience and self-compassion are essential throughout the process. Intermittent fasting is a journey that requires time and adjustment. Celebrate progress, no matter how small, and be compassionate towards yourself if you encounter setbacks. Consistency, persistence, and a positive mindset are key to success. By carefully building and adjusting the fasting schedule, intermittent fasting can become a transformative and rewarding practice for women over 50, promoting overall well-being and vitality.

Building a successful intermittent fasting schedule involves a comprehensive approach that includes understanding different fasting methods, preparing mentally and physically, and addressing common challenges. By selecting a fasting method that suits individual lifestyles and goals, staying hydrated, focusing on proper nutrition, getting adequate sleep, incorporating regular physical activity, and developing coping strategies for stress and social situations, women over 50 can create a sustainable and effective fasting schedule. With patience, flexibility, and a positive mindset, intermittent fasting can become a powerful tool for achieving health goals and enhancing overall quality of life.

5.1 Customizing Your Fasting Plan

"Take care of your body. It's the only place you have to live." - Jim Rohn.

This quote encapsulates the essence of customizing an intermittent fasting plan to suit individual needs. For women over 50, creating a personalized fasting schedule is not only about achieving specific health goals but also about honoring one's unique lifestyle, preferences, and routines. Customization ensures that the fasting plan is sustainable, enjoyable, and effective in promoting overall well-being.

The first step in customizing a fasting plan is to understand the different intermittent fasting methods and how they can be adjusted to fit various lifestyles. The 16/8 method, which involves fasting for 16 hours and eating during an 8-hour window, is highly adaptable and can be customized based on individual schedules. For instance, if someone prefers to eat dinner with their family, they might choose an eating window from noon to 8 p.m. On the other hand, if mornings are typically busy and breakfast is often skipped, an eating window from 10 a.m. to 6 p.m. might be more suitable. The flexibility of the 16/8 method allows for adjustments to meal timing that align with personal and social routines.

The 5:2 diet, which includes five days of regular eating and two non-consecutive days of reduced caloric intake, can also be tailored to fit different lifestyles. For those with a demanding workweek, choosing fasting days on less busy days, such as weekends, can make the plan more manageable. Alternatively, if weekends are filled with social events, fasting days could be scheduled during the week. This approach allows for flexibility while still providing the benefits of intermittent fasting.

Alternate-day fasting involves fasting every other day, which can be challenging but effective for some individuals. Customizing this method involves considering one's energy levels, work commitments, and social engagements. For example, if exercise is a regular part of the routine, it might be beneficial to schedule fasting days on rest days and eating days on workout days to ensure adequate energy levels. Additionally, planning fasting days around fewer demanding activities can help make the approach more sustainable.

Time-restricted eating, where the eating window is limited to a certain number of hours each day, offers a straightforward way to customize intermittent fasting. The eating window can be adjusted based on daily routines and preferences. For example, someone who enjoys a late dinner might choose a later eating window, such as 2 p.m. to 10 p.m. Conversely, if early breakfasts are preferred, an earlier window like 8 a.m. to 4 p.m. can be implemented. The key to success with time-restricted eating is consistency and finding an eating window that aligns with natural hunger patterns and daily schedules.

For those new to intermittent fasting, starting gradually and easing into the chosen method can be beneficial. Begin with a shorter fasting period and gradually extend it as the body adapts. For example, starting with a 12-hour fast and progressively increasing it to 14 or 16 hours can help minimize discomfort and make the transition smoother. This gradual approach allows the body to adjust to the new eating pattern and reduces the likelihood of experiencing hunger pangs or energy dips.

Incorporating flexibility into the fasting plan is crucial for long-term success. Life is dynamic, and there will be days when sticking to the fasting schedule might be challenging. Allowing for occasional flexibility, such as adjusting the eating window for special events or social gatherings, can help maintain a balanced and stress-free approach. The goal is to create a sustainable plan that fits seamlessly into one's lifestyle rather than feeling restrictive or burdensome.

Personal preferences and routines play a significant role in customizing an intermittent fasting plan. Consider daily activities, work schedules, exercise routines, and social commitments when designing the plan. For instance, if mornings are typically busy with work or family responsibilities, a later eating window might be more practical. Alternatively, if evenings are filled with social events or family dinners, an earlier eating window can accommodate these activities. The key is to find a balance that supports both health goals and lifestyle needs.

Sample fasting plans can provide a helpful starting point for customization. Here are a few examples tailored to different lifestyles:

For a busy professional:

- Fasting method: 16/8
- Eating window: 12 p.m. to 8 p.m.
- Meal schedule: Lunch at 12 p.m., afternoon snack at 3 p.m., dinner at 7 p.m.
- Tips: Prepare meals and snacks in advance to ensure healthy options are readily available during the eating window. Stay hydrated with water, herbal tea, or black coffee during the fasting period.

For an active individual with regular workouts:

- Fasting method: 16/8 or alternate-day fasting

- Eating window: 10 a.m. to 6 p.m. (16/8) or eating on workout days and fasting on rest days (alternate-day fasting)

- Meal schedule: Breakfast at 10 a.m., post-workout snack at 1 p.m., dinner at 5 p.m.

- Tips: Plan workouts during the eating window to ensure optimal energy levels and recovery. Include nutrient-dense foods to support exercise performance and muscle repair.

For someone with a social lifestyle:

- Fasting method: 5:2

- Fasting days: Tuesday and Thursday with 500-600 calorie intake

- Regular eating days: Monday, Wednesday, Friday, Saturday, and Sunday

- Meal schedule: Regular meals on non-fasting days, light meals on fasting days (e.g., vegetable soup, salads, lean protein)

- Tips: Plan social events on non-fasting days to allow for flexibility and enjoyment. Focus on nutrient-rich foods to maximize the benefits of fasting.

For a retiree with a flexible schedule:

- Fasting method: Time-restricted eating

- Eating window: 8 a.m. to 4 p.m.

- Meal schedule: Breakfast at 8 a.m., lunch at 12 p.m., afternoon snack at 3 p.m.

- Tips: Incorporate leisurely activities, such as morning walks or gardening, into the daily routine. Enjoy nutrient-dense meals that provide sustained energy throughout the day.

Mental preparation is an essential component of customizing an intermittent fasting plan. Setting clear, realistic goals and understanding the reasons for fasting can provide motivation and focus. Reflect on personal health goals, such as weight management, improved metabolic health, or enhanced energy levels, and how intermittent fasting can help achieve them. Keeping a journal to track progress, experiences, and adjustments can provide valuable insights and reinforce commitment.

Physical preparation involves ensuring the body is ready for the changes that intermittent fasting will bring. Gradually adjusting meal frequencies and sizes can help the body adapt to longer fasting periods. For instance, reducing snacking between meals and focusing on balanced, nutrient-dense meals can ease the transition. Staying well-hydrated is crucial during both fasting and eating periods. Drink plenty of water, and consider herbal teas, black coffee, and electrolyte-rich beverages to maintain hydration and support metabolic functions.

Proper nutrition during eating windows is vital for overall health and the success of the fasting plan. Focus on whole, unprocessed foods that provide essential nutrients, such as vitamins, minerals, and macronutrients. Include a variety of fruits, vegetables, lean proteins, healthy fats, and complex carbohydrates in meals. Prioritizing nutrient-dense foods not only supports overall health but also helps stabilize blood sugar levels, reduce cravings, and sustain energy.

Listening to the body's signals and responding appropriately is key to customizing an intermittent fasting plan. Pay attention to hunger and fullness cues and eat mindfully during eating windows. Avoid overeating or consuming high-calorie, low-nutrient foods out of fear of deprivation. Instead, focus on nourishing the body with wholesome foods that provide sustained energy and support overall well-being. Mindful eating practices, such as eating slowly, savoring each bite, and avoiding distractions, can enhance the dining experience and promote better digestion.

Quality sleep is a fundamental aspect of a successful intermittent fasting plan. Adequate sleep supports metabolic health, regulates hormones, and enhances overall well-being. Aim for 7-9 hours of sleep each night to ensure the body is well-rested and ready to adapt to the new eating pattern. Establishing a consistent sleep routine, such as going to bed and waking up at the same time each day, and creating a relaxing bedtime environment can promote restful sleep.

Regular physical activity complements intermittent fasting by supporting metabolic health, improving energy levels, and enhancing overall fitness. Incorporate a mix of aerobic exercises, strength training, and flexibility exercises into the routine. Be mindful of the timing and intensity of workouts, especially during fasting periods. Moderate-intensity exercises, such as walking, yoga, or light resistance training, can be performed during fasting windows, while more intense workouts may be better suited to eating windows to ensure optimal energy levels and performance.

Addressing common challenges and pitfalls is essential for customizing an intermittent fasting plan. The initial adjustment period may involve feelings of hunger, low energy, or irritability, which are typically temporary as the body adapts. To ease this transition, focus on staying hydrated, consuming nutrient-dense foods during eating windows, and incorporating stress-reduction techniques into daily routines. Social situations and cultural norms can also pose challenges, such as social gatherings or family events centered around food. Communicating fasting goals to friends and family and seeking their support can help navigate these situations. Alternatively, planning the fasting schedule around social events can allow for flexibility while maintaining commitment to intermittent fasting.

Emotional eating and stress can undermine the benefits of intermittent fasting. Developing coping strategies to manage stress and emotions, such as practicing mindfulness, engaging in physical activity, or seeking support from a therapist or counselor, can help address these challenges. Building a support network of friends, family, or a fasting community can provide encouragement and accountability, making the journey more enjoyable and sustainable.

Flexibility and willingness to adjust the fasting schedule as needed are important for maintaining long-term success. Be open to modifying the schedule based on individual needs and lifestyle changes. For example, if the chosen fasting method is not sustainable or causing undue stress, consider trying a different approach or adjusting the fasting and eating windows. The goal is to find a method that fits seamlessly into daily life and supports overall health and well-being.

Patience and self-compassion are essential throughout the process. Intermittent fasting is a journey that requires time and adjustment. Celebrate progress, no matter how small, and be compassionate towards yourself if you encounter setbacks. Consistency, persistence, and a positive mindset are key to success. By carefully customizing the fasting plan to suit personal preferences and routines, intermittent fasting can become a transformative and rewarding practice for women over 50, promoting overall well-being and vitality.

5.2 Adapting to Your Lifestyle

"Success is the sum of small efforts, repeated day in and day out." - Robert Collier. T

his quote is a reminder that integrating intermittent fasting into a busy lifestyle requires consistent, mindful adjustments rather than drastic changes. For women over

50, balancing work, family, and social commitments can seem daunting, but with thoughtful planning and flexibility, intermittent fasting can seamlessly become a part of daily life.

Intermittent fasting offers a variety of methods, allowing for a customizable approach that fits individual schedules. The 16/8 method, where one fasts for 16 hours and eats within an 8-hour window, is particularly popular due to its flexibility. For someone with a typical 9-to-5 job, a common strategy is to eat between noon and 8 p.m. This way, breakfast can be skipped, lunch can be eaten at work, and dinner can be enjoyed with family in the evening. Adjusting meal times slightly earlier or later can also accommodate different work shifts or personal preferences. The key is to find a consistent eating window that aligns with one's daily routine.

Family commitments often revolve around meals, making it essential to adapt fasting schedules without disrupting family time. For example, if family dinners are a cherished tradition, one could align the eating window to include dinner. Starting the fasting period after dinner ensures that family meals remain a joyful and integral part of daily life. Alternatively, incorporating smaller, nutrient-dense snacks within the eating window can help bridge any gaps and maintain energy levels for family activities.

Social commitments can also be seamlessly integrated into an intermittent fasting lifestyle. When attending social events, it's helpful to plan ahead. If an event falls outside the regular eating window, adjusting the fasting schedule for that day can provide the flexibility needed. For instance, shifting the eating window earlier or later by a few hours can accommodate a special dinner or celebration. Communicating with friends and family about fasting goals can foster understanding and support, making it easier to stick to the plan without feeling socially isolated.

Work commitments often pose a challenge for maintaining a fasting schedule, especially with irregular hours or frequent meetings. Planning meals and snacks in advance can help ensure that healthy, satisfying options are available during eating windows. Preparing lunch and snacks the night before or on weekends can save time and reduce the temptation to break the fast with less healthy options. Utilizing breaks to eat mindfully and staying hydrated throughout the day can also support energy levels and focus during fasting periods.

Staying flexible and adjusting the fasting schedule as needed is crucial for long-term success. Life is dynamic, and there will be times when strict adherence to a fasting plan is challenging. Recognizing that it's okay to adjust the plan temporarily can reduce stress and make intermittent fasting more sustainable. For example, during holidays or travel, the fasting schedule might need to be more flexible. Returning to the regular fasting routine once the event or trip is over can help maintain consistency without feeling deprived.

Mental preparation is equally important when adapting intermittent fasting to one's lifestyle. Setting realistic expectations and understanding that perfection is not required can make the journey more manageable.

Reflecting on personal health goals and the reasons for fasting can provide motivation and reinforce commitment during challenging times. Keeping a journal to track progress, experiences, and any necessary adjustments can offer valuable insights and foster a positive mindset.

Physical preparation involves ensuring the body is ready for the changes that intermittent fasting will bring. Gradually extending fasting periods can help the body adapt without significant discomfort. For instance, starting with a 12-hour fast and progressively increasing it to 14 or 16 hours can ease the transition. During eating windows, focusing on nutrient-dense foods that provide sustained energy can support overall health and make fasting periods more manageable.

Proper hydration is essential during both fasting and eating periods. Drinking plenty of water, herbal teas, and other non-caloric beverages can help maintain hydration and support metabolic functions. Staying hydrated also helps manage hunger and keeps energy levels stable throughout the day. For those who enjoy coffee, black coffee can be consumed during fasting periods without breaking the fast, providing an additional boost of energy and mental clarity.

Quality sleep is fundamental to the success of an intermittent fasting plan. Adequate sleep supports metabolic health, regulates hormones, and enhances overall well-being. Aiming for 7-9 hours of sleep each night can ensure the body is well-rested and ready to adapt to the new eating pattern. Establishing a consistent sleep routine, such as going to bed and waking up at the same time each day, and creating a relaxing bedtime environment can promote restful sleep.

Regular physical activity complements intermittent fasting by supporting metabolic health, improving energy levels, and enhancing overall fitness. Incorporating a mix of aerobic exercises, strength training, and flexibility exercises into the routine can be beneficial. Be mindful of the timing and intensity of workouts, especially during fasting periods. Moderate-intensity exercises, such as walking, yoga, or light resistance training, can be performed during fasting windows, while more intense workouts may be better suited to eating windows to ensure optimal energy levels and performance.

Addressing common challenges and pitfalls is essential for adapting intermittent fasting to one's lifestyle. The initial adjustment period may involve feelings of hunger, low energy, or irritability, which are typically temporary as the body adapts. To ease this transition, focus on staying hydrated, consuming nutrient-dense foods during eating windows, and incorporating stress-reduction techniques into daily routines. Social situations and cultural norms can also pose challenges, such as social gatherings or family events centered around food. Communicating fasting goals to friends and family and seeking their support can help manage these situations. Alternatively, planning the fasting schedule around social events can allow for flexibility while maintaining commitment to intermittent fasting.

Emotional eating and stress can undermine the benefits of intermittent fasting. Developing coping strategies to manage stress and emotions, such as practicing mindfulness, engaging in physical activity, or seeking support from a therapist or counselor, can help address these challenges. Building a support network of friends, family, or a fasting community can provide encouragement and accountability, making the journey more enjoyable and sustainable.

Flexibility and willingness to adjust the fasting schedule as needed are important for maintaining long-term success. Be open to modifying the schedule based on individual needs and lifestyle changes. For example, if the chosen fasting method is not sustainable or causing undue stress, consider trying a different approach or adjusting the fasting and eating windows. The goal is to find a method that fits seamlessly into daily life and supports overall health and well-being.

Patience and self-compassion are essential throughout the process. Intermittent fasting is a journey that requires time and adjustment. Celebrate progress, no matter how small, and be compassionate towards yourself if you encounter setbacks. Consistency, persistence, and a positive mindset are key to success. By carefully customizing the fasting plan to suit personal preferences and routines, intermittent fasting can become a transformative and rewarding practice for women over 50, promoting overall well-being and vitality.

By selecting a fasting method that suits individual lifestyles and goals, staying hydrated, focusing on proper nutrition, getting adequate sleep, incorporating regular physical activity, and developing coping strategies for stress and social situations, women over 50 can create a sustainable and effective fasting plan. With patience, flexibility, and a positive mindset, intermittent fasting can become a powerful tool for achieving health goals and enhancing overall quality of life.

CHAPTER SIX

NUTRITION FOR OPTIMAL HEALTH

"Let food be thy medicine and medicine be thy food."
- Hippocrates.

This ancient wisdom resonates even more profoundly in today's world, where nutrition plays a pivotal role in promoting health and well-being, especially for women over 50. As we jump into the realm of intermittent fasting as a solution, it becomes clear that this approach not only supports weight management but also enhances metabolic health, balances hormones, and fosters longevity.

Intermittent fasting (IF) has gained considerable attention for its potential health benefits beyond traditional dieting. For women over 50, who often face unique challenges related to hormonal changes, metabolism, and aging, IF offers a flexible and sustainable approach to achieving optimal health. By alternating periods of eating with periods of fasting, IF aligns eating patterns with natural metabolic rhythms, potentially enhancing nutrient absorption, insulin sensitivity, and cellular repair processes.

Understanding Intermittent Fasting Methods

One of the most popular IF methods is the 16/8 protocol, where individuals fast for 16 hours and consume all their calories within an 8-hour window. This method is particularly appealing due to its adaptability to daily routines. For instance, starting the eating window around noon and finishing it by 8 p.m. allows for skipping breakfast while still enjoying lunch and dinner with family or friends.

Integrating IF into Daily Life

Family and social dynamics often revolve around shared meals, making it essential to integrate IF without compromising these important social connections. Adjusting the fasting period to begin after dinner ensures participation in family dinners while maintaining the fasting schedule. Including nutrient-dense snacks within the eating window helps sustain energy levels during family activities and social engagements.

Managing Work Commitments

Balancing work commitments with IF requires strategic planning. Packing nutritious lunches and snacks in advance ensures healthy eating during the eating window, minimizing the temptation to break the fast with less healthy options. Hydration and mindful eating practices further support sustained energy and focus throughout the fasting period, enhancing productivity and overall well-being.

Flexibility and Adaptation

Flexibility is key to sustainable IF practice. Life's demands fluctuate, and there will be times when strict adherence to a fasting schedule is challenging. Allowing for temporary adjustments during holidays, travel, or special occasions reduces stress and promotes long-term adherence. Returning to the regular fasting routine afterward reinforces commitment and ensures consistency in health goals.

Mental Preparation

Preparing mentally for IF involves setting realistic expectations and understanding that adaptation takes time. Reflecting on personal health goals and motivations strengthens resolve, empowering individuals to persevere through initial challenges. Keeping a journal to track progress and experiences provides valuable insights and encourages a positive mindset, reinforcing the benefits of IF as part of a holistic approach to health.

Physical Readiness

Physical preparation complements mental readiness by ensuring the body can comfortably adapt to fasting periods. Gradually extending fasting durations allows for a smoother transition. Consuming nutrient-dense foods during eating windows supports overall health and enhances the effectiveness of IF in promoting metabolic health.

Hydration and Sleep

Hydration is crucial during both fasting and eating periods. Drinking ample water, herbal teas, and other non-caloric beverages supports metabolic functions and helps manage hunger throughout the day. Quality sleep is equally important for successful IF. Adequate rest supports metabolic processes, hormone regulation, and overall well-being, ensuring women over 50 are well-prepared to embrace the benefits of IF in their daily lives.

Incorporating Physical Activity

Regular physical activity complements IF by promoting metabolic health, improving energy levels, and enhancing overall fitness. Balancing aerobic exercises, strength training, and flexibility exercises supports comprehensive well-being. Adjusting workout intensity and timing relative to fasting periods optimizes energy expenditure and performance, maximizing the benefits of both IF and exercise.

Addressing Challenges

Navigating challenges inherent in IF requires awareness and proactive strategies. Initial adjustments may involve temporary sensations of hunger or fatigue as the body adapts to fasting periods. Prioritizing hydration, consuming nutrient-dense foods during eating windows, and integrating stress-reduction techniques into daily routines mitigate these challenges, promoting sustainable adherence to IF.

Emotional Well-Being

Emotional well-being is integral to sustained IF success. Developing coping strategies to manage stress and emotional eating behaviors enhances resilience and promotes positive outcomes. Engaging in mindfulness practices, seeking support from loved ones, or consulting with healthcare professionals fosters emotional resilience and strengthens commitment to long-term health goals.

Flexibility and Long-Term Success

Flexibility remains essential for maintaining long-term IF success. Adjusting fasting methods or modifying eating and fasting windows accommodates evolving lifestyles and ensures ongoing adherence to health goals.

6.1 Essential Nutrients for Women Over 50

"Let food be thy medicine and medicine be thy food." - Hippocrates.

This age-old adage underscores the profound impact of nutrition on our health, especially as we age. For women over 50, prioritizing essential nutrients through a balanced diet is crucial not only for maintaining health but also for supporting vitality and well-being. As we explore the vital nutrients that play a pivotal role in this stage of life, we sift into the significance of nutrient-dense foods and the benefits they offer within the context of intermittent fasting.

Key Nutrients for Women Over 50

Calcium: Essential for bone health, calcium becomes increasingly important as women age to mitigate the risk of osteoporosis and fractures. Dairy products, leafy greens like kale and collard greens, and fortified foods are excellent sources.

Vitamin D: Works in tandem with calcium to support bone health and immune function. Aging adults often have reduced ability to synthesize vitamin D from sunlight, making dietary sources like fatty fish (salmon, mackerel), egg yolks, and fortified foods essential.

Vitamin B12: Critical for neurological function and red blood cell production. With age, absorption of B12 from food decreases, highlighting the importance of consuming fortified cereals, meat, fish, and dairy products.

Folate (Folic Acid): Supports cell division and helps prevent neural tube defects in pregnancies. Green leafy vegetables, legumes, citrus fruits, and fortified grains are excellent sources.

Magnesium: Important for muscle and nerve function, blood sugar regulation, and bone health. Nuts, seeds, whole grains, and leafy green vegetables are rich sources of magnesium.

Omega-3 Fatty Acids: Promote heart health, reduce inflammation, and support brain function. Fatty fish (salmon, sardines), flaxseeds, chia seeds, and walnuts are abundant sources.

Potassium: Crucial for maintaining healthy blood pressure and muscle function. Bananas, potatoes, citrus fruits, and leafy greens are excellent sources of potassium.

Iron: Supports oxygen transport in the blood and energy production. Women over 50 may need more iron due to decreased absorption and blood loss. Lean meats, poultry, fish, beans, and fortified cereals are good sources.

Importance of Nutrient-Dense Foods

Nutrient-dense foods provide essential vitamins, minerals, and other beneficial compounds with relatively fewer calories. For women over 50, who may experience changes in metabolism and nutrient absorption, prioritizing nutrient density ensures optimal health and vitality. Incorporating these foods into balanced meals supports overall well-being and complements the benefits of intermittent fasting.

Building Balanced Meals

Balanced meals for women over 50 should emphasize:

Lean Proteins: Lean meats, poultry, fish, eggs, legumes, and tofu provide essential amino acids for muscle repair and immune function.

Whole Grains: Whole grains like quinoa, brown rice, oats, and whole wheat provide fiber for digestive health and sustained energy.

Healthy Fats: Sources such as avocados, nuts, seeds, and olive oil provide omega-3 and omega-6 fatty acids for heart health and cognitive function.

Colorful Fruits and Vegetables: Rich in vitamins, minerals, and antioxidants, fruits and vegetables support immune function and reduce the risk of chronic diseases.

Dairy or Dairy Alternatives: Low-fat dairy products or fortified plant-based alternatives provide calcium and vitamin D for bone health.

Integrating Nutrient-Dense Foods with Intermittent Fasting

Intermittent fasting enhances nutrient absorption and metabolic efficiency, making it a complementary approach to nutrient-dense eating for women over 50. By focusing on nutrient-rich foods during eating windows, individuals can optimize the benefits of both strategies. For instance, consuming calcium-rich dairy products or fortified alternatives during the eating window supports bone health, while omega-3 fatty acids from fatty fish promote heart health and cognitive function.

Practical Tips for Implementing Nutrient-Dense Eating

Meal Planning: Plan meals and snacks that incorporate a variety of nutrient-dense foods to ensure adequate intake of essential vitamins and minerals.

Portion Control: Practice mindful eating to avoid overconsumption and ensure balanced nutrient intake during eating windows.

Hydration: Stay hydrated with water and other non-caloric beverages throughout the day to support metabolic functions and overall health.

Supplementation: Consult with a healthcare provider about the need for supplements to address specific nutrient deficiencies common in women over 50.

Benefits Beyond Nutrition

Embracing a diet rich in essential nutrients not only supports physical health but also enhances cognitive function, mood stability, and overall quality of life for women over 50. Combined with intermittent fasting, which promotes metabolic health and cellular repair, nutrient-dense eating becomes a cornerstone of holistic well-being in this stage of life.

Prioritizing essential nutrients through nutrient-dense foods and balanced meals is fundamental for promoting health and vitality in women over 50. By understanding the roles of key nutrients and incorporating them into daily dietary habits, individuals can optimize health outcomes and support longevity. Intermittent fasting serves as a complementary approach, enhancing the benefits of nutrient-dense eating by promoting metabolic efficiency and cellular rejuvenation. Through mindful dietary choices and a commitment to holistic well-being, women over 50 can embrace a vibrant, fulfilling lifestyle supported by optimal nutrition and intermittent fasting.

6.2 Crafting Balanced Meals

"Let food be thy medicine and medicine be thy food." - Hippocrates. This timeless wisdom underscores the profound impact of nutrition on our health and well-being, especially as we age. Crafting balanced meals that are both nutritious and satisfying is essential for women over 50, supporting overall health, energy levels, and vitality. As we explore guidelines for meal composition, meal prep strategies, and portion control within the context of intermittent fasting, we uncover practical approaches to optimizing dietary habits for long-term well-being.

Guidelines for Creating Nutritious Meals

Incorporate Lean Proteins: Choose lean sources of protein such as poultry, fish, lean cuts of meat, tofu, and legumes. Protein is essential for muscle maintenance, immune function, and satiety, particularly important in supporting muscle mass and strength as we age.

Include Whole Grains: Opt for whole grains like quinoa, brown rice, oats, and whole wheat pasta. These provide fiber, vitamins, and minerals that support digestive health, regulate blood sugar levels, and provide sustained energy throughout the day.

Load Up on Colorful Vegetables: Aim to fill half of your plate with a variety of colorful vegetables. Vegetables are rich in antioxidants, vitamins, and minerals that support immune function, reduce inflammation, and promote overall health.

Incorporate Healthy Fats: Include sources of healthy fats such as avocados, nuts, seeds, olive oil, and fatty fishlike salmon. These fats are crucial for heart health, brain function, and absorption of fat-soluble vitamins like A, D, E, and K.

Choose Low-Fat Dairy or Dairy Alternatives: Opt for low-fat dairy products or fortified plant-based alternatives like almond milk or soy yogurt. These provide essential nutrients like calcium and vitamin D important for bone health.

Limit Added Sugars and Processed Foods: Minimize intake of foods high in added sugars, refined grains, and processed fats. These contribute to inflammation, weight gain, and may increase the risk of chronic diseases such as diabetes and cardiovascular disease.

Tips for Meal Prep

Plan Ahead: Take time to plan your meals for the week, considering your schedule and dietary goals. Planning helps ensure balanced nutrition and reduces the temptation to opt for less healthy, convenient options.

Batch Cooking: Prepare large batches of staple foods such as grains, proteins, and vegetables at the beginning of the week. This allows for quick assembly of meals throughout the week, saving time and promoting consistency in healthy eating.

Use Pre-cut and Frozen Ingredients: Utilize pre-cut vegetables, frozen fruits, and pre-cooked proteins to streamline meal preparation. These ingredients are convenient and retain their nutritional value, making meal prep less daunting.

Portion Control: Use portion control strategies such as measuring cups, plates, or containers to ensure appropriate serving sizes. This helps prevent overeating and supports weight management goals, particularly beneficial when practicing intermittent fasting.

Balance Macros: Aim for a balanced ratio of macronutrients (carbohydrates, proteins, and fats) in each meal to promote satiety and sustained energy. Adjust portion sizes based on individual energy needs and activity levels.

Incorporating Intermittent Fasting

Intermittent fasting enhances meal planning and portion control by defining specific eating windows, promoting mindful eating habits, and optimizing nutrient absorption. By aligning nutrient-dense meals with fasting periods, individuals can maximize the benefits of both approaches, supporting metabolic health, and promoting cellular repair.

Practical Meal Ideas

Breakfast: Greek yogurt with berries and nuts, whole grain toast with avocado and poached eggs, or a smoothie with spinach, banana, and protein powder.

Lunch: Quinoa salad with grilled chicken and mixed vegetables, lentil soup with whole grain bread, or a tuna salad wrap with whole wheat tortilla and leafy greens.

Dinner: Baked salmon with quinoa and roasted vegetables, tofu stir-fry with brown rice, or turkey meatballs with whole grain pasta and marinara sauce.

Snacks: Fresh fruit with a handful of nuts, vegetable sticks with hummus, or yogurt with granola.

Benefits of Balanced Meals Beyond Nutrition

Crafting balanced meals not only supports physical health but also enhances cognitive function, mood stability, and overall quality of life for women over 50. Combined with intermittent fasting, which promotes metabolic efficiency and cellular rejuvenation, balanced meal planning becomes a cornerstone of holistic well-being in this stage of life.

CHAPTER SEVEN

MEAL PLANNING AND RECIPES

Meal planning plays a crucial role in ensuring that women over 50 receive adequate nutrition while navigating the challenges and opportunities presented by intermittent fasting. By strategically organizing meals within defined eating windows, individuals can optimize nutrient intake, support metabolic health, and enhance overall well-being.

Benefits of Meal Planning

Meal planning offers numerous benefits beyond convenience. It helps individuals:

Promote Nutrient Balance: Plan meals that provide a balanced mix of carbohydrates, proteins, healthy fats, vitamins, and minerals essential for overall health and vitality.

Support Weight Management: Control portion sizes and calorie intake, facilitating weight loss or maintenance goals.

Save Time and Reduce Stress: Streamline grocery shopping and meal preparation, freeing up time for other activities and minimizing last-minute decisions.

Optimize Nutrient Timing: Coordinate meals with intermittent fasting schedules to maximize nutrient absorption and metabolic efficiency.

Principles of Effective Meal Planning

Set Goals and Priorities: Identify health goals such as improving heart health, managing blood sugar levels, or supporting bone density. Prioritize nutrient-dense foods that align with these objectives.

Consider Dietary Preferences and Restrictions: Tailor meal plans to accommodate dietary preferences, allergies, or medical conditions. Incorporate a variety of foods to ensure enjoyment and adherence.

Choose Nutrient-Dense Foods: Emphasize whole grains, lean proteins, fruits, vegetables, healthy fats, and dairy or dairy alternatives rich in essential nutrients. These foods provide sustained energy and support overall health.

Plan Balanced Meals: Aim for a mix of colors, textures, and flavors to enhance meal satisfaction. Include a variety of food groups in each meal to ensure comprehensive nutrition.

Prepare in Advance: Use batch cooking, meal prep techniques, and make-ahead recipes to streamline meal preparation and ensure nutritious meals are readily available during fasting and eating windows.

Practical Tips for Effective Meal Planning

Create a Weekly Meal Schedule: Outline meals for each day of the week, considering factors like work schedules, social engagements, and fasting windows.

Shop Wisely: Compile a grocery list based on planned meals and stick to it to avoid impulse purchases. Choose fresh, seasonal produce and minimally processed foods whenever possible.

Utilize Leftovers: Plan meals that yield leftovers for subsequent meals or snacks. Repurpose ingredients creatively to minimize waste and maximize nutritional value.

Include Variety: Rotate recipes and incorporate diverse cuisines and cooking methods to maintain interest and enjoyment. Experiment with new ingredients to expand culinary horizons.

Stay Hydrated: Include water, herbal teas, and other non-caloric beverages to stay hydrated throughout the day, supporting metabolic function and overall health.

SAMPLE MEAL PLANS AND RECIPES

Breakfast Ideas:

1. Greek Yogurt Parfait

- Greek yogurt topped with berries, nuts, and a drizzle of honey.

- Serve with whole grain toast or a small serving of granola.

2. Vegetable Omelette

- Two-egg omelette filled with spinach, tomatoes, and bell peppers.
- Serve with a side of whole grain toast or a slice of avocado.

Lunch Ideas:

1. Quinoa Salad with Chickpeas

- Quinoa mixed with chickpeas, cucumbers, cherry tomatoes, and feta cheese.
- Tossed with a lemon vinaigrette dressing and served over a bed of mixed greens.

2. Grilled Chicken Wrap

- Grilled chicken breast wrapped in a whole wheat tortilla with lettuce, tomato, avocado, and a light spread of hummus.

Dinner Ideas:

- Baked Salmon with Asparagus

- Salmon fillet seasoned with lemon, garlic, and herbs, baked until tender.

- Served with roasted asparagus and a side of quinoa or brown rice.

Vegetable Stir-Fry

- Mixed vegetables (broccoli, bell peppers, snap peas) stir-fried with tofu or shrimp in a light soy sauce and ginger sauce.

- Served over a portion of whole grain noodles or cauliflower rice.

Snack Ideas:

- Fresh Fruit with Nut Butter: Slices of apple or banana paired with almond or peanut butter for a satisfying snack rich in fiber and healthy fats.

- Trail Mix: A mix of nuts, seeds, and dried fruit for a portable, nutrient-dense snack.

- Smoothies: Blend spinach, berries, Greek yogurt, and a scoop of protein powder with water or almond milk for a refreshing and nutritious snack option.

Incorporating Intermittent Fasting

Intermittent fasting enhances the benefits of meal planning by establishing structured eating windows that support metabolic health and optimize nutrient absorption. By aligning nutrient-dense meals with fasting periods, individuals can promote cellular repair, improve insulin sensitivity, and enhance overall energy levels. Intermittent fasting also encourages mindful eating practices, promoting a deeper connection with hunger cues and food choices.

Meal planning is a valuable tool for women over 50 seeking to optimize nutrition and support overall health within the framework of intermittent fasting. By adopting strategic meal planning principles, incorporating nutrient-dense foods, and preparing meals in advance, individuals can achieve their health goals while enjoying varied and satisfying meals. Intermittent fasting complements these efforts by promoting metabolic efficiency and supporting cellular rejuvenation. Through thoughtful meal preparation and adherence to balanced nutrition, women over 50 can embrace a vibrant, fulfilling lifestyle supported by optimal nutrition and intermittent fasting.

7.1 Creating a Weekly Meal Plan

"Take care of your body. It's the only place you have to live." – Jim Rohn.

This quote encapsulates the essence of prioritizing health through mindful nutrition, especially as we age. Creating a weekly meal plan is a proactive approach that empowers women over 50 to optimize their nutritional intake while integrating the benefits of intermittent fasting. By strategically planning meals and snacks within defined eating windows, individuals can support metabolic health, enhance energy levels, and promote overall well-being.

Step-by-Step Guide to Planning Meals for the Week

Assess Your Nutritional Needs: Begin by evaluating your health goals, dietary preferences, and any specific nutritional requirements based on age or medical conditions. Consider consulting with a healthcare provider or nutritionist for personalized guidance.

Define Your Eating Windows: Determine the duration and timing of your fasting and eating windows. Common intermittent fasting methods include the 16/8 method (16 hours fasting, 8 hours eating) or the 5:2 method (regular eating for 5 days, restricted calories for 2 days).

Create a Weekly Calendar: Use a calendar or meal planning template to outline meals for each day of the week, considering factors such as work schedules, social commitments, and fasting periods. This visual aid helps organize meals and ensures variety.

Plan Balanced Meals: For each day, aim to include a mix of lean proteins, whole grains, fruits, vegetables, and healthy fats. Distribute these food groups across meals to achieve balanced nutrition and enhance meal satisfaction.

Incorporate Variety: Rotate recipes and ingredients to avoid monotony and ensure diverse nutrient intake.

Experiment with different cuisines, cooking methods, and seasonal produce to keep meals interesting.

Consider Meal Prep: Allocate time for meal preparation and batch cooking at the beginning of the week. Preparing components such as grains, proteins, and chopped vegetables in advance streamlines daily meal assembly.

Balance Macronutrients: Ensure each meal contains a balance of carbohydrates, proteins, and fats to support energy levels, satiety, and overall health. Adjust portion sizes based on individual energy needs and activity levels.

Sample Meal Ideas and Snack Options

Breakfast Ideas:

- Avocado Toast with Poached Egg: Whole grain toast topped with mashed avocado and a poached egg. Serve with a side of fresh fruit.
- Greek Yogurt Bowl: Greek yogurt topped with mixed berries, nuts, and a drizzle of honey. Accompany with a small serving of whole grain granola.

Lunch Ideas:

- Quinoa Salad with Grilled Chicken: Quinoa mixed with grilled chicken breast, cherry tomatoes, cucumber, feta cheese, and a lemon vinaigrette dressing. Serve over a bed of mixed greens.

- Vegetable Stir-Fry: Stir-fried mixed vegetables (broccoli, bell peppers, snap peas) with tofu or shrimp in a light soy sauce and ginger sauce. Enjoy with a side of brown rice or cauliflower rice.

Dinner Ideas:

- Baked Salmon with Asparagus: Salmon fillet seasoned with lemon, garlic, and herbs, baked until tender. Serve with roasted asparagus and quinoa.

- Turkey Meatballs with Whole Grain Pasta: Turkey meatballs in marinara sauce served over whole grain pasta. Accompany with a side of steamed green beans or a mixed salad.

Snack Options:

- Apple Slices with Almond Butter: Fresh apple slices paired with a tablespoon of almond butter for a satisfying and nutrient-dense snack.

- Trail Mix: A mix of nuts, seeds, and dried fruits for a portable and energizing snack option.

- Smoothie: Blend spinach, banana, berries, Greek yogurt, and a scoop of protein powder with water or almond milk for a refreshing and nutritious snack.

Integrating Intermittent Fasting

Integrating intermittent fasting into your weekly meal plan involves aligning meals with designated eating windows to optimize metabolic health and promote cellular repair. By practicing mindful eating during eating periods and staying hydrated throughout the fasting period, individuals can enhance the benefits of both nutrition and fasting strategies.

Benefits Beyond Nutrition

Beyond meeting nutritional needs, a well-planned weekly meal plan supports cognitive function, mood stability, and overall quality of life for women over 50. Regular meal planning fosters a sense of empowerment and control over dietary choices, promoting long-term adherence to healthy eating habits.

Creating a weekly meal plan is a proactive strategy for women over 50 seeking to prioritize health and well-being through balanced nutrition and intermittent fasting. By following a systematic approach to meal planning, incorporating diverse meal ideas and nutritious snacks, individuals can optimize nutrient intake, support metabolic health, and enhance overall vitality. Intermittent fasting enhances these efforts by promoting metabolic efficiency and cellular rejuvenation.

7.2 Delicious and Nutritious Recipes

Discovering delicious and nutritious recipes that align with intermittent fasting principles empowers women over

50 to nourish their bodies effectively while supporting metabolic health and overall well-being.

Nutrient-Rich Ingredients for Women Over 50

Leafy Greens: Rich in vitamins A, C, K, and folate, leafy greens like spinach, kale, and Swiss chard support bone health, immune function, and cognitive health.

Berries: Packed with antioxidants and fiber, berries such as blueberries, strawberries, and raspberries help combat oxidative stress, promote heart health, and support brain function.

Lean Proteins: Chicken breast, turkey, tofu, and legumes provide essential amino acids for muscle maintenance, immune support, and overall vitality.

Whole Grains: Quinoa, brown rice, oats, and whole wheat pasta offer fiber, B vitamins, and minerals like magnesium and selenium, promoting digestive health and sustained energy levels.

Healthy Fats: Avocado, nuts, seeds, and olive oil provide omega-3 fatty acids and monounsaturated fats crucial for heart health, cognitive function, and inflammation reduction.

Delicious and Nutritious Recipes

Breakfast Recipe: Greek Yogurt Parfait

Ingredients:

- 1 cup Greek yogurt
- 1/2 cup mixed berries (blueberries, strawberries)
- 1/4 cup granola (optional)
- Drizzle of honey or maple syrup (optional)

Instructions:

- In a glass or bowl, layer Greek yogurt, mixed berries, and granola.
- Repeat layers until ingredients are used, ending with a drizzle of honey or maple syrup if desired.
- Serve immediately and enjoy as a nutritious and satisfying breakfast option.

Lunch Recipe: Quinoa Salad with Chickpeas

Ingredients:

- 1 cup cooked quinoa
- 1/2 cup chickpeas, drained and rinsed
- 1/2 cucumber, diced
- 1/2 cup cherry tomatoes, halved
- 1/4 cup crumbled feta cheese
- Handful of fresh parsley, chopped
- Juice of 1 lemon
- 2 tablespoons olive oil
- Salt and pepper to taste

Instructions:

- In a large bowl, combine cooked quinoa, chickpeas, cucumber, cherry tomatoes, feta cheese, and parsley.
- In a small bowl, whisk together lemon juice, olive oil, salt, and pepper.
- Pour dressing over salad and toss gently to combine.

Serve chilled or at room temperature as a nutrient-packed lunch option.

Dinner Recipe: Baked Salmon with Asparagus

- Ingredients:

4 salmon fillets

1 bunch asparagus, trimmed

2 tablespoons olive oil

2 cloves garlic, minced

Juice of 1 lemon

Salt and pepper to taste

- Instructions:
- Preheat oven to 400°F (200°C). Line a baking sheet with parchment paper.
- Place salmon fillets on the prepared baking sheet. Arrange asparagus around the salmon.
- In a small bowl, whisk together olive oil, minced garlic, lemon juice, salt, and pepper.

- Drizzle half of the olive oil mixture over the salmon and asparagus.
- Bake for 12-15 minutes, or until salmon is cooked through and flakes easily with a fork.
- Remove from oven and drizzle remaining olive oil mixture over the cooked salmon and asparagus.
- Serve immediately as a flavorful and nutrient-rich dinner option.

Snack Recipe: Apple Slices with Almond Butter

- Ingredients:

1 apple, cored and sliced

2 tablespoons almond butter

Instructions:

- Arrange apple slices on a plate.
- Serve with almond butter for dipping or spreading.
- Enjoy as satisfying and nutritious snack rich in fiber and healthy fats.

Benefits of These Recipes for Women Over 50

These recipes are designed to provide essential nutrients, promote satiety, and support overall health for women over 50. By incorporating nutrient-rich ingredients and balanced meal compositions, these meals and snacks help maintain energy levels, support metabolic function, and contribute to long-term well-being.

Integrating Recipes with Intermittent Fasting

Aligning these recipes with intermittent fasting schedules enhances their benefits by promoting metabolic efficiency and optimizing nutrient absorption. By consuming nutrient-dense meals within defined eating windows, individuals can support cellular repair, improve insulin sensitivity, and enhance overall energy levels.

Exploring delicious and nutritious recipes tailored to the needs of women over 50 offers a pathway to optimal health and well-being. By incorporating nutrient-rich ingredients, balanced meal compositions, and mindful eating practices, individuals can nourish their bodies effectively while embracing the benefits of intermittent fasting. These recipes not only satisfy culinary preferences but also promote vitality, cognitive function, and overall quality of life. Through a commitment to wholesome nutrition and strategic meal planning, women over 50 can embark on a journey towards enhanced health and vitality supported by delicious and nutrient-packed recipes.

CHAPTER EIGHT

INCORPORATING EXERCISE AND MOVEMENT

This poignant reminder underscores the importance of prioritizing physical activity as a cornerstone of health, especially as women navigate the terrain of aging and embrace the benefits of intermittent fasting. Integrating exercise into daily routines not only enhances physical well-being but also complements the metabolic advantages of intermittent fasting, promoting vitality and longevity.

The Importance of Exercise for Women Over 50

Regular physical activity offers a multitude of benefits that are particularly relevant for women over 50. These include:

Maintaining Muscle Mass: Resistance training helps preserve muscle mass, which naturally declines with age. Strong muscles support joint health, posture, and overall mobility.

Enhancing Bone Health: Weight-bearing exercises such as walking, dancing, and strength training stimulate bone growth and density, reducing the risk of osteoporosis.

Supporting Metabolic Health: Exercise improves insulin sensitivity and enhances metabolic efficiency, which can complement the effects of intermittent fasting on blood sugar regulation and fat metabolism.

Promoting Heart Health: Aerobic activities like brisk walking, swimming, or cycling strengthen the heart muscle, improve circulation, and lower blood pressure, reducing the risk of cardiovascular disease.

Boosting Mood and Mental Health: Physical activity releases endorphins, neurotransmitters that promote feelings of well-being and reduce stress, anxiety, and depression.

Enhancing Cognitive Function: Regular exercise supports cognitive health by increasing blood flow to the brain, promoting neuroplasticity, and reducing the risk of cognitive decline.

Types of Exercise Recommended for Women Over 50

Aerobic Exercise

Aerobic exercise, also known as cardiovascular exercise, involves activities that increase heart rate and breathing. Examples include:

Brisk Walking: A low-impact exercise that can be done almost anywhere, promoting cardiovascular health and calorie burning.

Swimming: Gentle on the joints while providing a full-body workout, improving cardiovascular fitness and muscle tone.

Cycling: Whether indoors or outdoors, cycling improves leg strength and cardiovascular endurance, benefiting overall fitness.

Dancing: Engaging and enjoyable, dancing improves coordination, balance, and cardiovascular health.

Strength Training

Strength training involves using resistance to build muscle strength and endurance. Important exercises include:

Bodyweight Exercises: Such as squats, lunges, push-ups, and planks, which improve functional strength and stability.

Weight Machines: In a gym setting, machines provide controlled resistance for targeted muscle groups, supporting strength development.

Free Weights: Using dumbbells, kettlebells, or resistance bands, which offer versatility in resistance training exercises.

Flexibility and Balance Exercises

Flexibility and balance exercises help maintain joint mobility, prevent falls, and enhance overall physical function:

Yoga: Combines poses, breathing techniques, and meditation to improve flexibility, balance, and relaxation.

Tai Chi: A gentle martial art that emphasizes slow, flowing movements to enhance balance, coordination, and mental focus.

Pilates: Focuses on core strength, stability, and flexibility through controlled movements and breathing patterns

Incorporating Exercise with Intermittent Fasting

Integrating exercise into an intermittent fasting lifestyle requires thoughtful planning to maximize benefits while supporting fasting goals:

Timing Workouts: Schedule aerobic or strength training workouts during eating windows to optimize performance and recovery.

Hydration: Stay well-hydrated throughout the fasting period and during workouts to maintain energy levels and support muscle function.

Post-Workout Nutrition: Consume a balanced meal or snack containing protein and carbohydrates within the eating window to aid muscle repair and replenish glycogen stores.

Adaptation: Allow time for the body to adapt to exercise routines and fasting schedules, adjusting intensity and duration as needed.

Practical Tips for Getting Started

1. Set Realistic Goals:

Establish achievable goals based on current fitness levels, health considerations, and personal preferences.

2. Start Slowly and Progress Gradually:

Begin with low-impact activities and gradually increase intensity, duration, and frequency as fitness improves.

3. Mix It Up:

Incorporate a variety of exercises to prevent boredom, challenge different muscle groups, and promote overall fitness.

4. Listen to Your Body:

Pay attention to how your body responds to exercise and fasting. Adjust routines accordingly to avoid overexertion or discomfort.

5. Seek Professional Guidance:

Consult with a fitness trainer or healthcare provider to develop a safe and effective exercise program tailored to your needs and goals.

Benefits Beyond Physical Health

Embracing regular exercise as part of an intermittent fasting lifestyle offers holistic benefits that extend beyond physical health:

Enhanced Self-Esteem and Confidence: Achieving fitness goals and maintaining an active lifestyle promotes a positive self-image and sense of accomplishment.

Social Connection: Participating in group exercise classes or outdoor activities fosters social interaction and a sense of community.

Stress Reduction: Physical activity serves as a natural stress reliever, promoting relaxation and mental clarity.

Improved Sleep Quality: Regular exercise supports restful sleep, enhances sleep patterns, and contributes to overall well-being.

Incorporating exercise and movement into the daily routine of women over 50 is a pivotal step towards optimizing health and vitality. By embracing a variety of aerobic, strength training, flexibility, and balance exercises, individuals can enhance physical fitness, support metabolic health, and improve overall quality of life. When integrated with intermittent fasting, exercise synergistically promotes cellular rejuvenation, metabolic efficiency, and long-term well-being.

8.1 Finding the Right Exercise Routine

"Movement is a medicine for creating change in a person's physical, emotional, and mental states." - Carol Welch. This quote highlights the transformative power of exercise, especially when combined with the metabolic benefits of intermittent fasting. For women over 50, finding the right exercise routine is not just about staying active but optimizing health, vitality, and overall well-being through enjoyable and effective physical activities.

Benefits of Regular Physical Activity

Regular physical activity offers numerous benefits that are particularly valuable for women over 50, including:

Enhanced Muscle Strength and Endurance: Strength training exercises help maintain muscle mass, improve bone density, and support joint health.

Improved Cardiovascular Health: Aerobic exercises like walking, swimming, or cycling strengthen the heart muscle, improve circulation, and lower blood pressure.

Enhanced Metabolic Function: Exercise supports insulin sensitivity, promotes fat metabolism, and complements the metabolic benefits of intermittent fasting.

Mood Regulation: Physical activity stimulates the release of endorphins, reducing stress, anxiety, and symptoms of depression.

Enhanced Cognitive Function: Regular exercise supports cognitive health by increasing blood flow to the brain and promoting neuroplasticity.

Complementing Exercise with Intermittent Fasting

Integrating exercise with intermittent fasting enhances the benefits of both practices:

Improved Fat Utilization: Fasting primes the body to burn stored fat for energy, while exercise further enhances fat metabolism, supporting weight management and body composition.

Optimized Muscle Maintenance: Protein synthesis increases post-exercise, aiding muscle repair and maintenance, especially important for preserving muscle mass as we age.

Enhanced Cellular Repair: Both fasting and exercise promote cellular rejuvenation and autophagy, the process of clearing out damaged cells to support overall cellular health.

Balanced Energy Levels: Regular exercise during eating windows helps utilize nutrients effectively, sustaining energy levels throughout the day.

Selecting Enjoyable and Effective Exercises

1. Consider Personal Preferences:

Choose activities that you enjoy and look forward to, whether it's walking in nature, dancing to music, or practicing yoga. Enjoyment enhances adherence to the exercise routine.

2. Assess Physical Abilities:

Take into account current fitness levels and any health considerations. Consult with a healthcare provider or fitness professional to tailor exercises that are safe and appropriate.

3. Incorporate Variety:

Include a mix of aerobic, strength training, flexibility, and balance exercises to target different muscle groups, prevent boredom, and maximize overall fitness.

4. Adaptability and Accessibility:

Select exercises that can be easily integrated into daily life and adapted to varying schedules and environments. This may include home workouts, outdoor activities, or gym-based exercises.

5. Progress Gradually:

Start with low-impact activities and gradually increase intensity, duration, and frequency as fitness improves. This approach minimizes the risk of injury and allows for sustainable progress.

Examples of Effective Exercises for Women Over 50

Aerobic Exercises:

Brisk Walking: Improves cardiovascular fitness, strengthens leg muscles, and can be done almost anywhere.

Swimming: Provides a full-body workout while being gentle on the joints, promoting cardiovascular health and muscle tone.

Cycling: Enhances leg strength and cardiovascular endurance, suitable for outdoor or stationary cycling.

Strength Training Exercises:

Bodyweight Exercises: Such as squats, lunges, push-ups, and planks, improve functional strength and stability without requiring equipment.

Resistance Band Exercises: Offer resistance for muscle strengthening exercises, targeting specific muscle groups effectively.

Weight Training: Utilizing free weights or machines to increase muscle mass, improve bone density, and support metabolic health.

Flexibility and Balance Exercises:

Yoga: Enhances flexibility, promotes relaxation, and improves balance and posture through various poses and breathing techniques.

Tai Chi: Combines gentle movements and deep breathing to improve balance, coordination, and mental focus.

Pilates: Focuses on core strength, flexibility, and muscle control through controlled movements and mindful breathing.

Integrating Exercise Routine into Daily Life

To maintain consistency and maximize benefits, consider these practical tips for integrating exercise into daily routines:

Schedule Regular Exercise Sessions: Allocate dedicated time for exercise during eating windows, ensuring consistency and adherence to the routine.

Combine Activities: Incorporate physical activity into daily tasks, such as taking the stairs instead of the elevator, gardening, or walking meetings.

Stay Hydrated: Drink plenty of water before, during, and after exercise to maintain hydration and support optimal physical performance.

Prioritize Recovery: Allow time for rest and recovery between exercise sessions to prevent fatigue and support muscle repair and growth.

Finding the right exercise routine for women over 50 is a transformative journey towards enhancing physical health, mental well-being, and overall quality of life. By selecting enjoyable and effective exercises that complement the metabolic benefits of intermittent fasting, individuals can optimize muscle strength, cardiovascular health, and metabolic function. Embracing a diverse range of aerobic, strength training, flexibility, and balance exercises ensures holistic fitness while accommodating personal preferences and physical abilities.

8.2 The Role of Physical Activity in Fasting

"In every walk with nature, one receives far more than he seeks." - John Muir. This quote resonates deeply as we explore the symbiotic relationship between physical activity and intermittent fasting for women over 50. Understanding how exercise impacts fasting and vice versa is crucial for optimizing health, vitality, and overall well-being through integrated lifestyle practices.

The Impact of Exercise on Fasting

Physical activity influences fasting in several profound ways, enhancing its metabolic benefits and overall effectiveness:

Enhanced Fat Utilization: Exercise during fasting periods encourages the body to burn stored fat for energy more efficiently. This synergy supports weight management and promotes lean muscle preservation.

Improved Insulin Sensitivity: Regular exercise enhances insulin sensitivity, making cells more responsive to insulin and improving glucose metabolism. When combined with intermittent fasting, this effect can further stabilize blood sugar levels.

Promotion of Autophagy: Exercise stimulates autophagy, the cellular process of removing damaged or dysfunctional components. Intermittent fasting amplifies this process, promoting cellular rejuvenation and longevity

Accelerated Metabolism: Both exercise and fasting can boost metabolic rate temporarily. When integrated, they create a metabolic environment that supports fat loss and metabolic flexibility.

Optimized Muscle Maintenance: Protein synthesis increases post-exercise, aiding in muscle repair and maintenance. This is particularly beneficial for preserving muscle mass, which tends to decline with age.

The Role of Fasting in Exercise Performance

Intermittent fasting can influence exercise performance and recovery in ways that complement physical activity:

Enhanced Fat Adaptation: Fasting trains the body to rely on fat stores for energy, which can benefit endurance athletes and individuals engaged in prolonged aerobic activities.

Improved Energy Efficiency: During fasting periods, the body becomes more efficient at utilizing available energy sources, potentially enhancing endurance and stamina during workouts.

Post-Exercise Recovery: Consuming balanced meals or snacks during eating windows supports muscle repair, replenishes glycogen stores, and aids in recovery post-exercise.

Cognitive Benefits: Fasting has been shown to enhance cognitive function and mental clarity, which can positively impact focus and concentration during workouts.

Tips for Timing Workouts with Fasting Periods

Effective timing of workouts in relation to fasting periods can optimize performance, energy levels, and metabolic benefits:

1. Morning Workouts:

Before Eating Window: Engage in light to moderate aerobic exercises such as brisk walking or yoga before breaking the fast. This can help kickstart metabolism and enhance fat burning.

During Eating Window: Perform more intense workouts such as strength training or high-intensity interval training

(HIIT) to capitalize on post-exercise protein synthesis and nutrient utilization.

2. Afternoon or Evening Workouts:

Around Eating Window: Schedule workouts to coincide with the eating window for optimal fueling and recovery. This timing supports muscle repair and replenishes energy stores effectively.

Before Fasting Period: If fasting begins in the evening, consider exercising earlier in the day to ensure adequate post-workout nutrition and recovery.

3. Flexibility and Adaptation:

Listen to Your Body: Adjust workout timing based on personal energy levels, preferences, and daily schedules. Experiment with different timings to find what works best for your body and lifestyle.

Hydration: Stay well-hydrated before, during, and after workouts, especially during fasting periods, to support performance and recovery.

4. Consistency and Progression:

Gradual Adaptation: Start with shorter workouts and gradually increase duration and intensity as your body adapts to fasting and exercise routines.

Variety: Incorporate a variety of exercises to target different muscle groups, prevent overuse injuries, and maintain overall fitness and mobility.

Integrating Physical Activity into Daily Life

To maximize the benefits of exercise and fasting, consider these practical tips for integrating physical activity into daily routines:

Create a Routine: Establish a consistent schedule for workouts and fasting periods, aligning them with daily activities and responsibilities.

Multitasking: Combine exercise with daily tasks, such as walking or cycling for errands, taking active breaks during work, or participating in household chores that involve physical movement.

Social Engagement: Join exercise classes, walking groups, or fitness communities to stay motivated, socialize, and make physical activity a fun part of daily life.

In summary, understanding the dynamic interplay between exercise and intermittent fasting is key to optimizing health and well-being for women over 50. By leveraging the metabolic benefits of both practices, individuals can enhance fat metabolism, improve insulin sensitivity, and support muscle maintenance and recovery. Effective timing of workouts in relation to fasting periods can further amplify these benefits, promoting endurance, energy efficiency, and overall physical performance. Through consistency, adaptation, and a balanced approach to health, women over 50 can embrace a lifestyle that integrates exercise and intermittent fasting, fostering vitality, longevity, and a profound sense of well-being.

CHAPTER NINE

MANAGING STRESS AND EMOTIONAL WELL-BEING

"The greatest weapon against stress is our ability to choose one thought over another." - William James.

Stress management is a crucial aspect of maintaining overall well-being, especially for women over 50 navigating the complexities of life and health, alongside the transformative practice of intermittent fasting. Understanding how to effectively manage stress and support emotional health can significantly enhance the benefits of this lifestyle choice.

Understanding Stress and Its Impact

Stress is a natural response to challenges and demands, but prolonged or excessive stress can have detrimental effects on physical, mental, and emotional health. For women over 50, stressors such as caregiving responsibilities, health concerns, work pressures, and life transitions can be particularly significant. Intermittent fasting, with its metabolic and potential cognitive benefits, offers a unique opportunity to support stress resilience and emotional well-being.

The Role of Intermittent Fasting in Stress Management

Intermittent fasting influences stress management through several mechanisms:

Regulation of Hormones: Fasting can stabilize cortisol levels, the primary stress hormone, potentially reducing the physiological impact of chronic stress.

Enhanced Brain Function: Fasting promotes brain-derived neurotrophic factor (BDNF) production, which supports cognitive function and resilience against stress.

Improved Mood: Fasting may enhance mood regulation through neurochemical changes and increased serotonin production, which can positively impact emotional well-being.

Autophagy and Cellular Repair: Fasting activates cellular repair mechanisms like autophagy, which may contribute to overall resilience and health maintenance in the face of stress.

Strategies for Managing Stress and Enhancing Emotional Well-Being

1. Mindfulness and Relaxation Techniques:

Mindful Breathing: Practice deep breathing exercises to calm the mind and reduce physiological responses to stress.

Meditation: Incorporate mindfulness meditation to cultivate present-moment awareness and promote relaxation.

Yoga and Tai Chi: Engage in gentle movements and postures that promote relaxation, flexibility, and stress reduction.

2. Physical Activity:

Regular Exercise: Incorporate aerobic exercises, strength training, or yoga into your routine to release endorphins, improve mood, and reduce stress levels.

Nature Walks: Spend time outdoors in natural environments, which has been shown to reduce stress and enhance well-being.

3. Nutrition and Hydration:

Balanced Diet: Consume nutrient-dense foods rich in antioxidants, vitamins, and minerals to support overall health and resilience against stress.

Hydration: Stay adequately hydrated throughout the day to support cognitive function, mood stability, and overall well-being.

4. Social Support:

Maintain Connections: Foster relationships with friends, family, or support groups to share experiences, seek advice, and receive emotional support.

Join Communities: Engage in social activities or group activities that promote a sense of belonging and reduce feelings of isolation.

5. Sleep Quality:

Establish a Routine: Maintain consistent sleep-wake cycles to regulate circadian rhythms and support optimal sleep quality.

Create a Relaxing Environment: Prepare a calming bedtime routine, such as reading or listening to soothing music, to promote relaxation and improve sleep.

Integrating Stress Management with Intermittent Fasting

1. Routine and Consistency:

Structured Eating Windows: Plan meals and snacks during eating windows to ensure balanced nutrition and support stable energy levels throughout the day.

Mindful Eating: Practice mindful eating techniques to savor meals, enhance digestion, and promote a positive relationship with food.

2. Adaptability and Flexibility:

Adjustment Period: Allow time for the body to adapt to intermittent fasting, recognizing that initial adjustments may affect mood and energy levels temporarily.

Listen to Your Body: Pay attention to hunger cues, energy levels, and emotional responses to fasting, making adjustments as needed to support overall well-being.

3. Emotional Awareness and Self-Care:

Journaling: Keep a journal to reflect on thoughts, emotions, and experiences related to fasting and stress management, promoting self-awareness and emotional clarity.

Self-Compassion: Practice self-compassion and acceptance, acknowledging that challenges and setbacks are natural parts of the journey toward health and well-being.

Managing stress and supporting emotional well-being is essential for women over 50 integrating intermittent fasting into their lifestyles. By cultivating mindfulness, engaging in regular physical activity, nourishing the body with balanced nutrition, fostering social connections, and prioritizing quality sleep, individuals can enhance resilience against stress and promote overall health and vitality. Intermittent fasting, with its metabolic benefits and potential for cognitive enhancement, offers a complementary approach to stress management, supporting long-term well-being and a fulfilling life. Through intentional practices and a holistic approach to health, women over 50 can navigate life's challenges with resilience, grace, and a profound sense of self-care.

9.1 Techniques for Stress Reduction

"In today's rush, we all think too much, seek too much, want too much, and forget about the joy of just being." - Eckhart Tolle. This quote reflects the essence of mindfulness and the importance of embracing moments of calm amidst life's demands. For women over 50 navigating the intricacies of health and intermittent fasting, integrating stress reduction techniques and self-care practices is essential for fostering resilience and well-being.

Stress Reduction Techniques

Stress is a common part of life, but chronic stress can adversely affect physical and emotional health, making it crucial to incorporate effective stress reduction techniques into daily routines. Here are several techniques that can help women over 50 manage stress more effectively:

Mindfulness Practices:

Mindfulness involves paying attention to the present moment without judgment, which can significantly reduce stress and enhance overall well-being. Practices such as mindful breathing, body scans, and mindful walking can help cultivate awareness and promote relaxation

Meditation:

Meditation is a practice that involves focusing the mind and eliminating distractions, fostering inner peace and emotional balance. Guided meditation, mantra meditation, or mindfulness meditation can be particularly beneficial for reducing stress and promoting mental clarity.

Deep Breathing Exercises:

Deep breathing techniques, such as diaphragmatic breathing or box breathing, help activate the body's relaxation response, reduce muscle tension, and promote feelings of calmness and relaxation.

Progressive Muscle Relaxation (PMR):

PMR involves tensing and then relaxing different muscle groups systematically, helping to release physical tension and promote relaxation throughout the body.

Visualization:

Visualization techniques involve mentally imagining a peaceful place or scenario, which can help reduce stress, enhance mood, and promote feelings of well-being.

Importance of Self-Care and Relaxation

Self-care is essential for maintaining physical, emotional, and mental health, especially for women over 50 who may juggle multiple responsibilities and health concerns. Incorporating regular self-care practices promotes resilience and supports overall well-being:

Physical Self-Care:

Engaging in regular physical activity, such as walking, yoga, or dancing, not only improves physical health but also enhances mood and reduces stress levels.

Nutritional Self-Care:

Eating a balanced diet rich in nutrient-dense foods supports overall health and energy levels. During intermittent fasting, focusing on quality nutrition during eating windows is crucial for maintaining optimal health.

Sleep Hygiene:

Establishing a regular sleep routine and creating a relaxing bedtime environment can improve sleep quality, enhance cognitive function, and promote emotional well-being.

Social Connection:

Maintaining meaningful relationships and seeking social support from friends, family, or support groups can provide emotional comfort, reduce feelings of isolation, and promote overall well-being.

Hobbies and Leisure Activities:

Engaging in hobbies or activities that bring joy and fulfillment, such as reading, gardening, or creative pursuits, can reduce stress and enhance quality of life.

Stress Management and Intermittent Fasting

Integrating stress reduction techniques with intermittent fasting can enhance the overall effectiveness of both practices:

Mindful Eating:

Practicing mindful eating during eating windows can enhance the enjoyment of food, improve digestion, and promote a positive relationship with eating and fasting.

Hydration:

Staying well-hydrated throughout the day supports cognitive function, mood stability, and overall well-being during intermittent fasting.

Flexibility and Adaptability:

Being flexible with intermittent fasting schedules and listening to your body's cues can reduce stress and enhance the sustainability of fasting practices.

Individuals can manage stress effectively, support emotional health, and enhance the benefits of intermittent fasting. Through intentional practices and a holistic approach to health, women over 50 can navigate life's challenges with grace, resilience, and a profound sense of self-care.

9.2 The Connection Between Mind and Body

"Your body hears everything your mind says." - Naomi Judd. This quote underscores the profound connection between our thoughts, emotions, and physical well-being. For women over 50 embarking on the journey of intermittent fasting, understanding and nurturing this mind-body connection is crucial for overall health and vitality.

The Relationship Between Emotional Well-Being and Physical Health

Emotional well-being significantly impacts physical health, influencing everything from immune function to longevity. Research has shown that positive emotional states can enhance resilience against illness and promote longevity, while chronic stress and negative emotions can weaken immune function and increase the risk of chronic diseases. For women over 50, who may be navigating life transitions, health challenges, and the adjustments of intermittent fasting, nurturing emotional well-being becomes even more essential.

Strategies for Maintaining a Positive Mindset

Maintaining a positive mindset can foster resilience, enhance overall health, and complement the benefits of intermittent fasting. Here are strategies to cultivate and sustain a positive outlook:

Gratitude Practice:

Cultivating gratitude through daily practices, such as keeping a gratitude journal or reflecting on blessings, can shift focus from challenges to sources of joy and appreciation.

Positive Affirmations:

Using positive affirmations, such as "I am strong and resilient," "I embrace change with grace," or "I trust in my body's wisdom," can reinforce self-confidence and a positive self-image.

Mindfulness Meditation:

Engaging in mindfulness meditation practices, which involve observing thoughts and sensations without judgment, promotes present-moment awareness and reduces stress levels.

Physical Activity:

Regular exercise, such as walking, yoga, or dancing, releases endorphins and neurotransmitters that enhance mood and reduce feelings of anxiety or depression.

Social Connection:

Maintaining meaningful relationships and engaging in social activities fosters a sense of belonging, support, and emotional well-being.

Nutritional Support:

Consuming a balanced diet rich in nutrients supports brain health and mood stability, optimizing emotional well-being during intermittent fasting.

Creative Expression:

Engaging in creative pursuits, such as painting, writing, or music, provides an outlet for emotions and promotes a sense of fulfillment and joy.

Integrating Emotional Well-Being with Intermittent Fasting

Integrating strategies for emotional well-being with intermittent fasting can enhance overall health and well-being:

Stress Management: Practicing stress reduction techniques, such as deep breathing exercises or progressive muscle relaxation, supports emotional balance during fasting periods.

Mindful Eating: Approaching meals with mindfulness and gratitude enhances enjoyment, digestion, and nutritional absorption.

Hydration: Staying hydrated throughout the day supports cognitive function, mood stability, and overall well-being during intermittent fasting.

Nurturing the connection between mind and body is vital for women over 50 navigating the challenges and benefits of intermittent fasting. By prioritizing emotional well-being through practices like gratitude, mindfulness, physical activity, and social connection, individuals can enhance resilience, support physical health, and optimize the transformative effects of intermittent fasting.

CHAPTER TEN

SUSTAINING LONG-TERM SUCCESS

"Success is not final, failure is not fatal: It is the courage to continue that counts." - Winston Churchill.

This quote encapsulates the essence of sustaining long-term success with intermittent fasting—a journey of persistence, adaptation, and commitment to health and well-being. For women over 50 embracing intermittent fasting, maintaining sustainable practices is crucial for reaping lasting benefits and enjoying a vibrant life.

Understanding Long-Term Success with Intermittent Fasting

Intermittent fasting has gained popularity for its potential health benefits, including weight management, metabolic health improvement, and longevity. However, sustaining these benefits over the long term requires a balanced approach that considers individual needs, lifestyle factors, and health goals.

Key Strategies for Long-Term Success

1. Personalized Approach

Every individual is unique, and what works for one person may not necessarily work for another. Tailoring intermittent fasting approaches to personal preferences, health conditions, and daily routines increases the likelihood of long-term adherence and success.

2. Consistency and Routine

Establishing a consistent fasting schedule and meal routine helps regulate metabolism, optimize hormone levels, and support digestive health. Consistency also fosters habit formation, making intermittent fasting easier to maintain over time.

3. Nutrient-Dense Eating

During eating windows, prioritizing nutrient-dense foods, such as fruits, vegetables, lean proteins, whole grains, and healthy fats, provides essential vitamins, minerals, and antioxidants. This supports overall health, energy levels, and mitigates nutrient deficiencies that can impact well-being.

4. Hydration

Staying well-hydrated throughout the day supports cognitive function, metabolism, and digestion during intermittent fasting. Consuming water, herbal teas, and other non-caloric beverages helps maintain hydration and enhances overall well-being.

5. Physical Activity

Incorporating regular physical activity complements intermittent fasting by supporting muscle mass maintenance, metabolism, and cardiovascular health. Choosing activities that are enjoyable and sustainable ensures long-term adherence and overall fitness.

6. Sleep Quality

Prioritizing adequate sleep duration and quality promotes hormone balance, cognitive function, and overall well-being. Establishing a bedtime routine, creating a conducive sleep environment, and practicing relaxation techniques enhance sleep quality during intermittent fasting.

7. Mindful Eating Practices

Practicing mindful eating, such as savoring each bite, chewing slowly, and listening to hunger cues, enhances digestion, promotes satiety, and fosters a positive relationship with food during intermittent fasting.

8. Social Support and Accountability

Engaging with supportive friends, family members, or online communities provides encouragement, motivation, and accountability on the intermittent fasting journey. Sharing experiences, challenges, and successes fosters a sense of camaraderie and reinforces long-term commitment.

Overcoming Challenges and Adapting to Change

Navigating challenges and adapting to life changes are integral to sustaining long-term success with intermittent fasting:

Travel and Social Events: Planning ahead, adjusting fasting schedules as needed, and making mindful food choices can help maintain consistency during travel or social gatherings.

Plateaus and Setbacks: Recognizing that occasional plateaus or setbacks are natural parts of the journey allows for adjustments in fasting approaches, meal composition, or physical activity to support continued progress.

Health Considerations: Consulting healthcare providers and nutritionists ensures that intermittent fasting practices align with individual health needs, such as managing chronic conditions, medications, or nutritional requirements.

Embracing a Holistic Approach to Well-Being

Embracing a holistic approach that integrates physical, emotional, and social well-being enhances the sustainability and effectiveness of intermittent fasting:

Emotional Well-Being: Practicing stress reduction techniques, fostering positive relationships, and engaging in activities that promote joy and fulfillment support mental health alongside intermittent fasting.

Educational Resources: Staying informed about current research, nutritional guidelines, and practical tips empowers individuals to make informed decisions and adapt intermittent fasting practices for long-term success.

sustaining long-term success with intermittent fasting for women over 50 involves a commitment to personalized approaches, consistency, nutritious eating, regular physical activity, adequate sleep, and mindful practices. By prioritizing holistic well-being, embracing flexibility, and navigating challenges with resilience, individuals can cultivate lasting health benefits and enjoy a vibrant, fulfilling life with intermittent fasting as a cornerstone of their wellness journey.

12.1 Making Intermittent Fasting a Lifestyle

"Success is not the key to happiness. Happiness is the key to success. If you love what you are doing, you will be successful." - Albert Schweitzer.

This quote resonates with the idea that integrating intermittent fasting into daily life can be a rewarding journey when approached with passion and commitment. For women over 50, embracing intermittent fasting as a lifestyle choice involves understanding its benefits, adapting routines, and fostering consistency over time.

Understanding Intermittent Fasting as a Lifestyle Choice

Intermittent fasting is more than a diet—it's a pattern of eating that alternate between periods of fasting and eating. This approach has gained popularity for its potential health benefits, including weight management, improved metabolic health, and enhanced longevity. For women over 50, these benefits can be particularly significant, supporting overall health and well-being as they navigate life's transitions and health considerations.

Integrating Intermittent Fasting into Daily Life

1. Choosing the Right Fasting Protocol

Selecting a fasting protocol that aligns with personal preferences, health goals, and lifestyle is crucial for long-term adherence. Common methods include the 16/8 method, where eating occurs within an 8-hour window, or alternate-day fasting, where fasting periods alternate with regular eating days. Experimenting with different approaches helps find the most sustainable option.

2. Establishing a Consistent Routine

Consistency is key to making intermittent fasting a habit. Establishing a consistent eating window and fasting schedule helps regulate metabolism, optimize hormone levels, and support digestive health. This routine also simplifies meal planning and enhances overall dietary adherence.

3. Balancing Nutrient-Dense Meals

During eating windows, prioritizing nutrient-dense foods such as vegetables, fruits, lean proteins, whole grains, and healthy fats provides essential nutrients and supports overall health. Balanced meals help maintain energy levels, promote satiety, and minimize cravings during fasting periods.

4. Hydration and Non-Caloric Beverages

Staying hydrated throughout the day is essential for overall health and well-being during intermittent fasting. Drinking water, herbal teas, and other non-caloric beverages can help curb hunger, support metabolic functions, and maintain hydration levels.

5. Mindful Eating Practices

Practicing mindful eating, such as savoring each bite, chewing slowly, and listening to hunger cues, enhances digestion, promotes satiety, and fosters a positive relationship with food. Mindfulness during meals supports overall dietary adherence and enjoyment.

Maintaining Balance and Consistency

1. Stress Management

Integrating stress management techniques, such as meditation, deep breathing exercises, or yoga, supports emotional well-being and reduces stress levels during intermittent fasting. Managing stress enhances overall resilience and supports long-term adherence.

2. Physical Activity

Incorporating regular physical activity complements intermittent fasting by supporting metabolic health, maintaining muscle mass, and enhancing overall fitness. Choosing activities that are enjoyable and sustainable promotes consistency and supports overall well-being.

3. Quality Sleep

Prioritizing adequate sleep duration and quality supports hormone balance, cognitive function, and overall well-being. Establishing a bedtime routine and creating a conducive sleep environment enhances sleep quality during intermittent fasting.

4. Social Support and Accountability

Engaging with supportive friends, family members, or online communities provides encouragement, motivation, and accountability on the intermittent fasting journey. Sharing experiences, challenges, and successes fosters a sense of community and reinforces long-term commitment.

Adapting to Life Changes and Challenges

1. Flexibility in Fasting Patterns

Being flexible with fasting schedules allows for adjustments during special occasions, travel, or unexpected events. Flexibility promotes sustainability and reduces stress associated with rigid dietary patterns.

2. Continuous Learning and Adaptation

Staying informed about nutrition, health research, and intermittent fasting best practices empowers individuals to make informed decisions and adapt their approach over time. Continuous learning supports long-term success and promotes overall well-being.

Through commitment, adaptation, and a holistic approach to health, intermittent fasting can become a rewarding and sustainable lifestyle choice for women over 50, supporting long-term health, wellness, and longevity.

12.2 Building a Supportive Community and Network

"Alone, we can do so little; together, we can do so much." - Helen Keller. This quote underscores the power of community in achieving common goals, including adopting and maintaining intermittent fasting as a lifestyle choice. For women over 50, cultivating a supportive network can provide encouragement, motivation, and shared experiences that enhance the journey toward better health and well-being.

Benefits of Having a Support System

1. Encouragement and Motivation

A supportive community offers encouragement during both challenges and successes encountered along the intermittent fasting journey. Sharing progress, tips, and motivational stories fosters a sense of camaraderie and inspires individuals to stay committed to their health goals.

2. Accountability and Commitment

Being part of a community promotes accountability, as members hold each other responsible for maintaining fasting routines and making healthy choices. Accountability partners or groups help reinforce commitment and reduce the likelihood of falling back into old habits.

3. Shared Knowledge and Resources

Communities provide a wealth of knowledge and resources related to intermittent fasting, nutrition, meal planning, and overcoming common challenges. Members can share practical tips, recipes, and research findings that support informed decision-making and enhance dietary adherence.

4. Emotional Support and Understanding

Navigating dietary changes can be emotionally challenging at times. A supportive network offers empathy, understanding, and a safe space to discuss feelings, setbacks, and successes without judgment. Emotional support strengthens resilience and promotes a positive mindset throughout the intermittent fasting journey.

Tips for Finding and Building a community

1. Join Online Forums and Social Media Groups

Platforms like Facebook groups, Reddit communities, and specialized forums provide opportunities to connect with individuals who share similar health goals and interests. Engaging in discussions, asking questions, and sharing experiences can foster meaningful connections and valuable support networks.

2. Attend Local Meetups and Workshops

Local meetups, workshops, or seminars focused on intermittent fasting, nutrition, and wellness offer opportunities to meet like-minded individuals in person. These events provide a supportive environment for sharing insights, learning from experts, and building relationships within the community.

3. Participate in Fitness Classes or Groups

Joining fitness classes, walking groups, or exercise clubs tailored for older adults can introduce you to individuals who prioritize health and well-being. These settings encourage physical activity while fostering friendships and mutual encouragement among participants.

4. Form Accountability Partnerships

Pairing up with a friend, family member, or online buddy who is also practicing intermittent fasting creates a personal accountability partnership. Regular check-ins, shared goals, and mutual support reinforce commitment and motivation to stick to fasting routines.

5. Contribute Positively to the Community

Actively contributing to the community by sharing insights, offering support to others, and celebrating collective achievements strengthens relationships and fosters a sense of belonging. Being a positive influence within the community enhances personal growth and enriches the overall experience of intermittent fasting.

Nurturing a Supportive Environment

1. Be Open to Learning and Growth

Remain open to learning from others' experiences and perspectives within the community. Embrace new ideas, strategies, and approaches to intermittent fasting that align with personal preferences and health goals.

2. Express Gratitude and Appreciation

Acknowledging and expressing gratitude for the support received from community members cultivates a positive atmosphere and strengthens interpersonal connections. Recognizing the impact of shared encouragement and guidance fosters a supportive and uplifting environment.

3. Celebrate Milestones and Achievements

Celebrate personal milestones, achievements, and breakthroughs within the community. Recognizing progress, no matter how small, reinforces motivation and inspires others to continue pursuing their health goals with determination and optimism.

In conclusion, building a supportive community and network plays a pivotal role in integrating intermittent fasting into daily life for women over 50. By fostering encouragement, accountability, shared knowledge, and emotional support, communities empower individuals to navigate challenges, embrace healthy habits, and sustain long-term success. Through active participation, openness to learning, and nurturing positive relationships, women over 50 can cultivate a supportive environment that enhances their well-being and enriches their intermittent fasting journey. By harnessing the power of community, individuals can achieve lasting health benefits and enjoy the journey towards a healthier, more fulfilling lifestyle.

APPENDICES

APPENDIX A: FREQUENTLY ASKED QUESTIONS

As you embark on your journey with intermittent fasting, you may encounter various questions and uncertainties. This appendix aims to address common queries to support your understanding and confidence in implementing intermittent fasting solutions tailored for women over 50.

Q: What is intermittent fasting (IF)?

Intermittent fasting is an eating pattern that alternates between periods of eating and fasting. It does not prescribe specific foods but rather focuses on when to eat them. This approach has gained popularity for its potential health benefits, including weight management, improved metabolic health, and cellular repair processes.

Q: Is intermittent fasting safe for women over 50?

Yes, intermittent fasting can be safe and beneficial for women over 50 when approached thoughtfully and with consideration of individual health conditions. It's essential to consult with a healthcare provider before starting IF, especially if you have underlying medical conditions or take medications that may be affected by fasting.

Q: What are the different methods of intermittent fasting?

There are several methods of intermittent fasting, including:

16/8 method: Involves daily fasting for 16 hours, with an 8-hour eating window.

5:2 method: Involves eating normally for five days of the week and restricting calorie intake to 500-600 calories on two non-consecutive days.

Alternate-day fasting: Involves alternating between days of normal eating and very low-calorie intake or fasting.

Q: How can intermittent fasting benefit women over 50?

Intermittent fasting may offer several benefits for women over 50, including:

Weight management: IF can help with weight loss and maintenance by reducing calorie intake and enhancing fat burning.

Metabolic health: IF may improve insulin sensitivity, reduce inflammation, and support healthy cholesterol levels.

Cellular repair: Fasting triggers cellular repair processes and enhances autophagy, which may contribute to longevity and overall health.

Q: Can intermittent fasting help with menopause symptoms?

Some women find that intermittent fasting helps manage symptoms associated with menopause, such as weight gain and hormonal fluctuations. However, individual responses may vary, and it's essential to monitor how IF affects your symptoms and overall well-being.

Q: What should I eat during the eating window of intermittent fasting?

During the eating window, focus on nutrient-dense foods that support overall health and well-being. Include a balance of lean proteins, whole grains, fruits, vegetables, and healthy fats. Avoid processed foods, sugary snacks, and excessive amounts of refined carbohydrates.

Q: How do I stay hydrated while fasting?

Staying hydrated is crucial during intermittent fasting. Drink plenty of water throughout the day, and consider incorporating herbal teas or flavored water for variety. Avoid sugary beverages and excessive caffeine intake, especially during fasting periods.

Q: What if I feel hungry or fatigued during fasting periods?

It's normal to experience hunger or fatigue, especially when starting intermittent fasting. Listen to your body and consider adjusting your fasting schedule or meal timing to better suit your needs. Incorporating nutrient-dense foods and staying hydrated can also help manage hunger and maintain energy levels.

Q: Should I exercise while intermittent fasting?

Yes, incorporating regular physical activity is beneficial and complements intermittent fasting. Choose exercises that you enjoy and that align with your fitness level. Aim for a combination of cardiovascular exercises, strength training, and flexibility exercises to support overall health and well-being.

Q: How long should I try intermittent fasting before expecting results?

Results from intermittent fasting can vary depending on individual factors such as age, health status, and adherence to the fasting protocol. It may take several weeks to months to notice significant changes in weight, metabolic health, or other health markers. Patience and consistency are key to experiencing the potential benefits of intermittent fasting.

APPENDIX B: ADDITIONAL RESOURCES AND READING

Exploring intermittent fasting for women over 50 opens up a world of possibilities for enhancing health and well-being. This appendix provides a curated list of resources and recommended reading to further support your journey into intermittent fasting and holistic health.

Websites and Online Resources:

The Obesity Code Podcast: Hosted by Dr. Jason Fung, this podcast discusses various aspects of fasting, insulin resistance, and metabolic health.

Diet Doctor: Provides evidence-based guides, meal plans, and recipes for intermittent fasting and low-carb diets.

Harvard Health Publishing: Offers articles and resources on intermittent fasting, health benefits, and practical tips for implementation.

Scientific Articles and Research:

PubMed: Search for research articles on intermittent fasting and its effects on metabolic health, aging, and chronic disease prevention.

Journal of Nutrition and Metabolism: Access peer-reviewed studies and reviews on intermittent fasting and its impact on various health markers.

Online Communities and Forums:

Reddit - r/intermittentfasting: Engage with a community of individuals practicing intermittent fasting, share experiences, and seek advice.

Facebook Groups: Join groups dedicated to intermittent fasting for women over 50, where members share tips, recipes, and support.

Health Apps:

MyFitnessPal: Track food intake, monitor fasting windows, and set personalized health goals.

Zero: A fasting tracker app that helps monitor fasting periods, track progress, and access resources on intermittent fasting.

Nutrition and Recipe Resources:

Cookbooks: Explore cookbooks focused on healthy recipes suitable for intermittent fasting, emphasizing nutrient-dense meals.

Healthy Eating Blogs: Follow blogs that specialize in nutritious meal ideas, meal planning tips, and dietary recommendations for intermittent fasting.

APPENDIX C: GLOSSARY OF TERMS

This glossary provides definitions of key terms and concepts related to intermittent fasting and women's health, aimed at enhancing your understanding and clarity as you explore this transformative health practice.

1. Autophagy: A natural process where cells remove and recycle damaged components, promoting cellular health and longevity. Autophagy is stimulated during fasting periods.

2. Circadian Rhythm: The body's internal clock that regulates various physiological processes, including sleep-wake cycles and metabolism. Intermittent fasting can influence circadian rhythms.

3. Insulin Resistance: A condition where cells become less responsive to insulin, leading to elevated blood sugar levels. Intermittent fasting may improve insulin sensitivity over time.

4. Ketosis: A metabolic state where the body uses fat for fuel instead of carbohydrates. Ketosis can occur during extended fasting periods or low-carbohydrate diets.

5. Metabolic Syndrome: A cluster of conditions including high blood pressure, high blood sugar, excess body fat around the waist, and abnormal cholesterol levels. Intermittent fasting may help reduce risk factors for metabolic syndrome.

6. Resting Metabolic Rate (RMR): The number of calories the body burns at rest to maintain basic physiological functions. Intermittent fasting may influence RMR.

7. Sirtuins: Proteins involved in regulating cellular health, metabolism, and longevity. Some research suggests intermittent fasting may activate sirtuins.

8. Time-Restricted Eating (TRE): A form of intermittent fasting where eating is restricted to a specific window of time each day, typically 8-12 hours.

9. Thermogenesis: The process of heat production in the body, often associated with metabolic processes and calorie burning. Intermittent fasting can influence thermogenesis.

10. Hormesis: The phenomenon where exposure to mild stressors (like fasting) results in adaptive responses that improve resilience and health outcomes.

11. Glycogen: A form of glucose stored in muscles and the liver for energy use. Fasting depletes glycogen stores, prompting the body to use fat for energy.

12. Macronutrients: Nutrients required by the body in large amounts: carbohydrates, proteins, and fats.

Balancing macronutrients is important for overall health during intermittent fasting.

13. Micronutrients: Essential vitamins and minerals required in smaller amounts for various physiological functions. Adequate intake of micronutrients is crucial during intermittent fasting.

14. Electrolytes: Minerals such as sodium, potassium, and magnesium that conduct electrical impulses in the body. Maintaining electrolyte balance is important during fasting.

15. Time Under Tension (TUT): A principle in exercise where muscles are kept under constant strain during movements, promoting muscle growth and strength.

16. Leptin: A hormone produced by fat cells that regulates appetite and energy balance. Intermittent fasting may influence leptin levels.

17. Ghrelin: A hormone produced in the stomach that stimulates hunger. Ghrelin levels typically rise before meals and decrease after eating.

18. Macronutrient Ratio: The proportion of carbohydrates, proteins, and fats in a diet. Adjusting macronutrient ratios can optimize outcomes during intermittent fasting.

19. Fasting Mimicking Diet (FMD): A diet designed to mimic the effects of fasting while still allowing some food intake, typically low in calories and carbohydrates.

20. Hormonal Balance: The optimal state where hormones are produced and regulated in appropriate amounts to support bodily functions and health.

CONCLUSION

Throughout history, the pursuit of health and longevity has been intertwined with the rhythms of life and the resilience of the human spirit. As we've explored in "Intermittent Fasting Solutions for Women Over 50: Transform Your Health," the journey towards optimal well-being is not just a matter of shedding pounds or slowing aging—it's about embracing a lifestyle that nurtures vitality and celebrates the wisdom of experience.

In the words of Hippocrates, "Let food be thy medicine and medicine be thy food." This ancient wisdom resonates deeply in the realm of intermittent fasting, where the deliberate modulation of eating patterns empowers women over 50 to reclaim control over their health destinies. The benefits extend far beyond physical transformation; they encompass a profound rejuvenation of body, mind, and spirit.

From understanding the science behind fasting to customizing schedules that fit diverse lifestyles, each chapter has served as a compass, guiding you through the nuances of this transformative practice. We've explored how intermittent fasting enhances metabolic flexibility, supports hormonal balance, and fosters cellular repair—essential pillars for thriving in the golden years.

Moreover, we've deeply explained the tortuous of nutrition, emphasizing the importance of nutrient-dense foods and balanced meals to complement fasting routines. We've shared practical meal plans, delicious recipes, and insights into optimizing exercise regimens to synergize with fasting benefits. Stress reduction techniques and mindfulness practices have been highlighted as vital tools for nurturing holistic well-being.

As you embark on your intermittent fasting journey, remember that it is not a sprint but a sustainable path towards vitality and longevity. The flexibility inherent in fasting methods allows you to tailor your approach to suit your unique preferences and daily rhythms. Whether it's embracing a time-restricted eating window or exploring fasting mimicking diets, each step contributes to your holistic transformation.

In closing, this book is not merely a guide but a companion on your quest for optimal health. It empowers you to savor life's moments with renewed energy and vitality, celebrating the wisdom and resilience that come with age. As you implement these principles into your daily life, remember that every small change contributes to a profound transformation—one that honors your body's innate ability to heal and thrive.

Let this journey be a testament to your strength and commitment to living your best life. Shed pounds, slow aging, boost energy, enhance well-being, and savor life—because your health journey is a testament to the power of resilience and the beauty of embracing change.

9 798333 210366 7